Perineal Trauma at Childbirth

Khaled M.K. Ismail
Editor

Perineal Trauma at Childbirth

Springer

Editor
Khaled M.K. Ismail
University of Birmingham
Birmingham, United Kingdom

ISBN 978-3-319-14859-5 ISBN 978-3-319-14860-1 (eBook)
DOI 10.1007/978-3-319-14860-1

Library of Congress Control Number: 2017932803

Printed on acid-free paper

This Springer imprint is published by Springer Nature
The registered company is Springer International Publishing AG
The registered company address is: Gewerbestrasse 11, 6330 Cham, Switzerland

Preface

In 2011, I was very privileged to meet a group of clinicians who share my clinical and academic interest. Without much debate or deliberation, the Perineal Trauma **P**revention, **E**ducation, **E**valuation, **R**epair and **S**canning (PEERS) group was conceived. This collaboration has enabled us to share good practice, publish collaboratively, run training workshops and along the way learn a lot from each other. To date, the PEERS group has conducted 5 full and 8 taster workshops in 11 countries spanning four continents. This textbook is the most recent challenge that the PEERS group, unanimously, agreed to take on board.

Perineal trauma at the time of childbirth affects hundreds of thousands of women in Europe and millions worldwide every year. A repair for such trauma is one of the commonest procedures undertaken in medicine. However, there are a few issues that are quite peculiar about this subject. It is an area of clinical practice that falls between two subspecialties (maternal medicine and uro-gynaecology), is assessed and repaired by two independent professions (obstetricians and midwives) and its complications managed by a large multidisciplinary team. Accordingly when planning the chapters for this book, we had these issues in mind and invited authors beyond the PEERS group to ensure that there is multidisciplinary input from leading clinicians in those fields. This book is also written and edited with both obstetricians and midwives in mind as target audience. Indeed all the authors of this book are committed to both multiprofessional training and service delivery.

There is high-level evidence demonstrating that proper assessment and repair of perineal trauma can significantly improve outcomes for women. However, nothing beats trauma prevention when it comes to long-term outcomes, particularly for higher grades of perineal trauma. The PEERS group is very keen on the dissemination of this aspect of care and indeed has dedicated several chapters in this book to highlight what practitioners can do to reduce risk of perineal trauma, obstetric anal sphincter injuries, wound complications and postnatal urinary incontinence. In addition to prevention, we present several aspects related to perineal trauma and its management including, a historic perspective, anatomy and physiology, clinical assessment, pelvic floor imaging, perineal mapping, methods and materials for repair and a framework for implementation of evidence into practice. The chapters within this book feed into each other and are interlinked. Nevertheless, each chapter covers a succinct topic and could be read on its own.

I feel honoured to be given the opportunity to edit this book. Apart from the enjoyment I had whilst reading about a clinical topic that I am very passionate about, it gave me time to reflect on several aspects: first, how little we know about something that is so common; second, how much we know that is not translated to actual care that would make a real difference; thirdly, how many of the challenges and difficulties that we face are, in fact, similar despite our perceived differences and last but not least how much women have endured over the ages and continue to do so.

I hope you enjoy reading this book as much as I enjoyed editing it.

University of Birmingham
Birmingham, UK

Khaled Ismail

Acknowledgements

The PEERS group who has created this reference work comprises a multiprofessional interdisciplinary team of clinical academics from different countries (currently all in Europe) who have a shared interest in the field of prevention and management of childbirth-related perineal trauma. Our group believes that structured training is key to facilitate the implementation of evidence into practice. Each member of our team has a vast and varied experience in delivering practical training in our area of interest in different settings and healthcare services.

PEERS has been running non-profit workshops since 2011 aimed at spreading evidence-based practice and building multiprofessional capacity with the ultimate goal of improving childbirth-related perineal outcomes for women globally.

Current PEERS Group Core Members:

Khaled Ismail – UK (Chair).

Vladimir Kalis – Czech Republic.

Katariina Laine – Norway.

Jan Willem de Leeuw – Netherlands.

Renaud de Tayrac – France.

Sari Raisanen – Finland.

Contents

Chapter 1
Perineal Trauma: A Historical and International Perspective

Christine Kettle and Khaled Ismail

Abstract Review of historical literature confirms that perineal injury has occurred during childbirth throughout the ages and that various methods and material were used by accoucheurs in an attempt to restore the integrity of severely traumatised tissue. Perineal stitching following childbirth was advocated in ancient writings on midwifery and obstetrics, however the procedure was not routinely practiced.

Women remained the prominent figure during confinements in the early centuries and male physicians or barber-surgeons were only called in as a last resort if problems occurred. During the eighteenth century the introduction of forceps together with episiotomy to facilitate difficult deliveries had a major impact on the extent of perineal trauma and its subsequent repair. Furthermore, women were encouraged to deliver in a more supine position rather than upright so the perineum was more accessible and the full extent of perineal trauma sustained could be assessed. During this period more attention was made to minimising perineal trauma and various methods including supporting the perineum and applying pressure to the vertex to prevent rapid expulsion were implemented. By the end of the nineteenth century practitioners were advised to suture all perineal trauma. However, it was not until the early twentieth century that local anaesthetic was advocated to ease the pain prior to performing and suturing episiotomies. In the UK, midwives did not receive any formal training until the late eighteenth century and it was not until the late twentieth century that midwives were permitted to undertake perineal suturing.

"May the lessons of the past be a guide to the future"

C. Kettle (✉)
Faculty of Health Sciences, Staffordshire University, Stoke-on-Trent, UK
e-mail: C.Kettle@staffs.ac.uk

K. Ismail
University of Birmingham, Birmingham, UK
e-mail: k.ismail@bham.ac.uk

K.M.K. Ismail (ed.), *Perineal Trauma at Childbirth*,
DOI 10.1007/978-3-319-14860-1_1

Keywords Childbirth • Historical • Perineal trauma • Man midwives • Ancient writings • Assessment • Classification • Non-suturing • Suturing • Perineal integrity and training

Introduction

Perineal trauma sustained during childbirth is not a new phenomenon as review of historical literature from 2050 BC to the 1900 AD confirms that women have suffered injury throughout the centuries. In fact, the earliest case of severe perineal injury sustained during childbirth was observed in the mummy of Henhenit. She was Nubian woman, approximately 22 years of age, and was thought to be a queen or a dancer in the court of King Mentuhotep of Egypt 2050 BC ([9, 18, 29], p. 15). Derry [9] observed that Henhenit's pelvis was an abnormal shape and that there was rupture of the vagina into the bladder, which may have been due to cephalopelvic disproportion occurring at the time of parturition and probably resulted in her early death.

This chapter will include review of ancient writings relating to perineal repair, factors contributing to the main causes of perineal trauma, assessment and classification, non-suturing, protecting the perineum, methods used to restore perineal integrity and training issues.

Ancient Writings Relating to Perineal Repair

As far back as early civilisation it has been tradition for labouring women to be attended by female '*midwives*', men were excluded from the birth chambers and the secrets of their profession were closely guarded. As a consequence very little information regarding normal childbirth was handed down in writing because '*women*' were usually uneducated and incapable of recording their experiences. The early writings on pregnancy and labour compiled by Hippocrates (born 460 BC) contributed very little to midwifery practice, probably due to the fact that physicians had very little scientific knowledge of the mechanisms of normal childbirth ([36], p. 2).

At the beginning of the second century Soranus, a Greek physician and distinguished writer on obstetrics and gynaecology, wrote on the subject of childbirth ([43], p. 15). One of his manuscripts, known as '*De Morbis Mulierium*', was the first textbook to be written for midwives and this became the principal midwifery treatise of ancient times and continued to be important throughout the next 1,500 years ([18], p. 72; [36], p. 2). Soranus's writings on obstetrics and gynaecology formed the foundation of many midwifery and obstetric textbooks that followed.

During the medieval period the standard text on obstetrics and gynaecology was based on a series of Latin works known as '*Trotula*' after its author ([12], p. 11; [43], p. 26). Trotula was thought to be a female physician or midwife who graduated from the famous Medical School of Salerno in Italy during the eleventh century. However, Towler and Bramall [43] suggest that Trotula (*Madame Trotte de Salerne*) may have been male who assumed female identity, as '*it would have been offensive to women for men to interest themselves in such matters*'. Graham [18] also supported this theory.

It would appear that '*Trotula*' was based on the original work of Soranus and throughout the text the '*midwife*' is instructed to deal with obstetric complications whilst the '*doctor*' addressed only gynaecological problems ([43], p. 27). Only two chapters deal with obstetric conditions and very little is mentioned about normal labour and delivery. '*Trotula*', was translated from the original Latin version into English during the fourteenth and fifteenth centuries. The manuscript was part of the Sir Hans Sloane medical manuscript collection (thirteenth to seventeenth century), which is now held at the British Library (Index number Sloane MS 2463).

The first English midwifery textbook to be printed was entitled '*The Byrthe of Mankynde*'. This was translated from '*De Morbis Mulierium*' by Richard Jonas and was published by Thomas Raynalde in 1540 (cited in [12], p. 11; [37], p. 14). The title was changed to '*The Woman's Boke*' in later editions. It is interesting to note that stitching of perineal trauma was advocated in all of these ancient writings on midwifery and obstetrics ([18], p. 121, [43], p. 27).

In the '*The Byrthe of Mankynde*' if a woman had a '*complete*' perineal tear, the midwife was instructed to wash the '*parts*' with '*butter and wine*' and to... "*sowe to geder yat pece that is broken with a silken threde with a quarell* [square sided] *nedell in thre places or on foure and sithen do pitche on a softe lynnen cloth and leye it to ye prevy members*" (cited in [36], p. 5). Following this procedure a linen dressing was applied to the wound and kept in position for 7 days, during which time the midwife was instructed to "*let her eten and drynken but litell and keep her well from cold and from etes and drynkes that might maken her eny coughe*" (cited in [18]).

Despite the fact that '*midwives*' were advised to stitch '*complete*' perineal tears following childbirth, it would appear that this procedure was not routinely practiced. Eccles [12] suggested that the reasons for not suturing might be due to either "*resistance on part of the patient or squeamishness on the part of the midwife*". Hence, '*The Byrthe of Mankynde*' recommended an alternative method of perineal repair, whereby pieces of linen cloth were stuck to each side of the perineal wound and then stitched together... "*take two lyttell peces of lynnen cloth, eche of the length of the wounde, and in bredth two fyngers brode: spred the lyttell clothes with some faste cleauynge plaster the which wyll cause the clothes to stycke fast where they shalbe set, then fasten them the one on the one syde of the ryfte, the other on the other side, so that nothyng appeare betwene the peces of lynnen in the myddes of them, but onely the clefte and ryfte of the wounde in the breadthe of a strawe, then this done, sowe these sydes of lynnen together close as before I bed you to sowe the skynne: and when they be thus styched to gether, laye a lyttell lyquyd pytche vpon the seme: and this done the lappes and sydes of the wounde vender the lynnen plaster wyll grow to gether agayne and heale, and then may ye remove your plasters*" (cited in [12], p. 105–106).

Factors Contributing to the Cause of Perineal Trauma

Insight into the cause and extent of perineal trauma sustained during childbirth was provided by the writings of '*man-midwife*' Percivall Willughby (1596–1685). He developed an interest in midwifery following his apprenticeship to a barber-surgeon and practised in Derby, Stafford and London. Willughby utilised his theoretical knowledge and practical skills to educate midwives not to interfere with the normal process of childbirth. During the time that Willughby practiced, it was common for women to deliver in a more upright position on birthing stools, with the '*private parts*' covered so that the midwife or accoucheur could not view the external genitalia during delivery thus maintaining modesty ([37], p. 12). However, at the first sign of labour, the attending midwife would try to manually dilate the cervix and stretch the vagina, which caused swelling to the genitalia and perineal injury ([12], p. 106).

Delivering babies remained mainly 'women's work' during the seventeenth century and families relied on skillful 'midwives' to safely deliver babies, however male physicians or barber-surgeons were called in, as a last resort, to assist if the midwife failed to deliver the baby. Sometimes he would have to dismember and extract the fetus with crochet hooks and knives to save the life of the mother, however, more often than not, these instruments caused considerable perineal injury and fistulae between the rectum, vagina and bladder. Any attempt made to repair this type of trauma often failed and the surviving victims of these traumatic births were reduced to a life of misery with '*weakness*', '*prolapsed organs*', vulval '*itching*' and no control over the bladder or bowels ([17], p. 232; [37], p. 43).

During this period of time, the Chamberlen brothers played a leading role in midwifery and a new technical advance emerged to revolutionise the management of difficult births. They became very successful as 'man- midwives' and they were invited to serve royalty. In a treatise on midwifery, Hugh Chamberlen claimed that his family had designed an instrument (the obstetric forceps) that could bring about a safe delivery, which was kept secret for more than 100 years. In order to maintain secrecy, the forceps were carried into the birthing room in a lined box and would only be used once everyone was out of the room and the mother was blindfolded or the baby was delivered under drapes. Once the secret was divulged, forceps were modified and used more widely during the eighteenth century, however there use remained controversial.

During the eighteenth century the introduction of forceps together with episiotomy to facilitate difficult deliveries had a major impact on the extent of perineal trauma and its subsequent repair. The primary repair of the episiotomy would quite often be unsuccessful but this was thought to be better than having a tear, which may have extended through into the rectum leaving the woman incontinent of faeces [37].

Episiotomy

According to the literature, Sir Fielding Ould was the first to describe the procedure of making a cut (perineotomy) into the perineum and he recommended that it should be performed in cases where the external vaginal opening was so tight that labour was dangerously prolonged [34]. At first this procedure was performed very rarely in emergencies as a last resort.

It was more than 100 years later when the procedure was reported in the United States of America by Taliaferro who described cutting a small mediolateral episiotomy to facilitate delivery in a young eclamptic woman [39].

Obstetricians only came to favour the procedure after publications by two American obstetricians [8, 35] which stated that perineotomy, was of 'extreme value in diminishing danger of death and injury to the first born' and should be performed routinely to shorten the second stage of labour; preserve the integrity of the pelvic floor and forestall uterine prolapse. DeLee redefined childbirth as pathogenic in nature and the perineum became a vulnerable site for surgical intervention [8].

By the 1930s, most American Hospitals had accepted episiotomy (perineotomy) as a routine procedure but it was not so widely used in Britain until the 1950s when childbirth became increasingly medicalised [42]. Episiotomy rates in the United Kingdom steadily increased until, by the 1970s it was as high as 91 % in some hospitals, [41]. This widely used obstetric procedure was introduced without substantial scientific evidence to support either its benefits or risks and its efficacy became the centre of controversy. Some argued that the procedure actually reduced the incidence of severe perineal trauma and prevented over stretching of the pelvic floor muscles which could lead to long-term problems such as stress incontinence and uterine prolapse [11, 16]. Others argued that episiotomy caused more pain, weakened the pelvic floor structures, interfered with breast-feeding and increased sexual problems [19, 27]. Major variations in current national rates may in itself indicate uncertain justification for this practice [1].

Classification and Assessment of Perineal Trauma

During the middle ages, women delivered in upright positions and their private parts were hidden under clothing as it was improper to cast one's eyes on the '*genitalia*', therefore little would be known regarding the full extent of trauma sustained. During the eighteenth century women were encouraged to deliver in a more supine position so that the perineum was more accessible and subsequent damage could be seen [15].

In 1897, Jellett described laceration of the perineum as "*one of the commonest accidents occurring in midwifery*" and stated that "*it occurs far more frequently than is supposed; as, unless it be looked for with care, it may not be noticed*". He also defined perineal trauma into two classifications:

a. *Complete: the laceration extends right through the perineal body into the rectum*
b. *Incomplete: the laceration involves the perineal body alone*

(Jellett [25], p. 234)

In the early twentieth century, DeLee reiterated the importance of thoroughly examining the perineum after delivery and wrote in his book for obstetric nurses that ….. '*of more importance are the tears of the pelvic floor, which are hard to find and are usually overlooked by the general practitioner. When the perineum is torn deeply, the anus and rectum may be laid open. This is a sad accident, as the woman may thus lose control of the bowel. Immediate repair of the injury should be made'* ([7], p. 33). He also described three degrees of perineal lacerations: *'first, through the fourchette; second, to, but not through the sphincter of the anus; and the third degree, through the anus into the rectum'* ([7], p. 118). This was similar to the definition of perineal tears that was used in the England up until the twenty-first century.

Non-suturing of Perineal Trauma

The controversy regarding the best management of perineal trauma, relating to suturing versus non-suturing, has continued throughout the centuries.

Prior to the seventeenth century, unless the perineum was severely torn the majority of trauma sustained during childbirth was left to heal naturally aided by ointments, some of which consisted of "*oil of worms and foxes with a little blind whelp, well boiled*" (cited in [12], p. 105). Herman [23] advised that tears would generally heal if the "*patient be kept clean with her legs tied together*" and that "*if the sides of the tear, is not perfect, the only result is that the vaginal orifice remains enlarged*". Even when severe perineal trauma was sutured, the failure rate was very high probably as a result of infection due to poor hygiene and lack of aseptic techniques. Puerperal fever was prolific due to "*interference in the birth canal*" by midwives and accoucheurs with "*unwashed hands and instruments*" and many women died as a result of this ([12], p. 129).

William Smellie, a London surgeon, and '*man-midwife*' (1697–1763) did not advise suturing the ruptured perineum except when the trauma was severe, because the stitches were inclined to cut through the tissue and were thought to be unnecessary [36]. Some practitioners including Willughby thought that it was not advisable to attempt to suture perineal trauma, even if it was severe and had extended into the rectum, as the '*rift*' would facilitate easier childbirth during subsequent deliveries. Whereas, French '*man-midwives*' of the mid-sixteenth century, such as La Vauguion and Pare, advocated stitching, even though the scar may complicate the next delivery, because they thought that "*the excrements coming that way*" from the women would disgust the husband and she would not be "*fit for his caresses*" (cited in [12]).

In 1904, DeLee wrote that …. ' *still it is also true that sometimes the perineum will tear like wet blotting-paper, and no skill can save it. In communities where the above notion is prevalent, the physician is often tempted to neglect the repair of lacerations of the perineum, as he will acquire a reputation of "tearing his women". His neighbour does not have lacerations because he does not put in so many "stitches". The nurse may do much to assist the conscientious physician by explaining to the family the frequency of injuries to the pelvic floor and the necessity for their repair'* ([7], page 118).

In the mid twentieth century, Magdi [29] reported that the incidence of perineal trauma at his hospital in Cairo was 24 % in primips as compared to 2 % in multips.

He associated this remarkably low rate of perineal injury among multiparous women to the fact that many of them had sustained damage during previous deliveries, which "*being attended by a midwife, was left unsutured*".

Magdi stated that it was a "*lamentable fact that midwives are in the habit of ignoring perineal trauma and neither practising nor calling for suturing to be performed*". Indeed, it would appear that the modern trend of midwives supporting a policy of non-suturing perineal trauma following childbirth is not a new concept.

Throughout the ages it is apparent that attempts were made to repair severe perineal trauma, using various methods and materials but as stated by Magdi [29] they were usually unsuccessful and "*the profession fell back to the helpless postural treatment*". Up until the late nineteenth century, women with severe perineal damage were confined to bed for up to 6 weeks and nursed on their side with their legs tied together to encourage healing by secondary intention [29].

Protecting the Perineum

Throughout the ages midwives have been instructed to support the perineum with a pad while the head is advancing to prevent severe perineal trauma. Soranus of Ephesus, in the second century, and Trotula, in the eleventh century, documented evidence of this practice [32, 40].

During the eighteen century, more attention was given to preventative methods to preserve the integrity of the perineum, which possibly developed as a result of the difficulties encountered in repairing severe perineal trauma. Harvie [22] wrote that '*were the delivery left to nature, the perineum would generally be torn at the time when the head of the child protrudes through the os externum, particularly at the birth of a first or second child*'. He also documented that …. '*the preservation the perineum being of the greatest consequence ought to be principally attended to by midwives; and this I think may be best done by observing the following rules, the importance of which experience had taught me*'. He then instructs the midwife to apply the palm of the hand against the perineum with '*proper force*' during the contraction in order to allow the fetal head to advance slowly and prevent tearing. He concluded by stating that… '*who ever attends to these rules, and puts them in practice with patience, will most certainly prevent the fatal consequences which hurrying a delivery to often produces*' [22].

In 1855 a German obstetrician named Ritgen, described a manoeuvre used during the second stage of labour to minimise perineal trauma. The accoucheur was instructed to reach for the fetal chin between the woman's anus and coccyx and to pull it anteriorly and at the same time the fingers of the other hand was placed on the fetal occiput to control the speed of the delivery and keep the head flexed (Fig. 1.1). The original manoeuvre was performed between contractions.

This was later modified and was performed during contractions in the second stage of labour and was first described in the 14th edition of Williams Obstetrics in 1971.

A similar technique was described by Solomon Bender (consultant obstetrician and gynaecologist – Chester) in his book titled 'Obstetrics for Pupil Midwives' ([3],

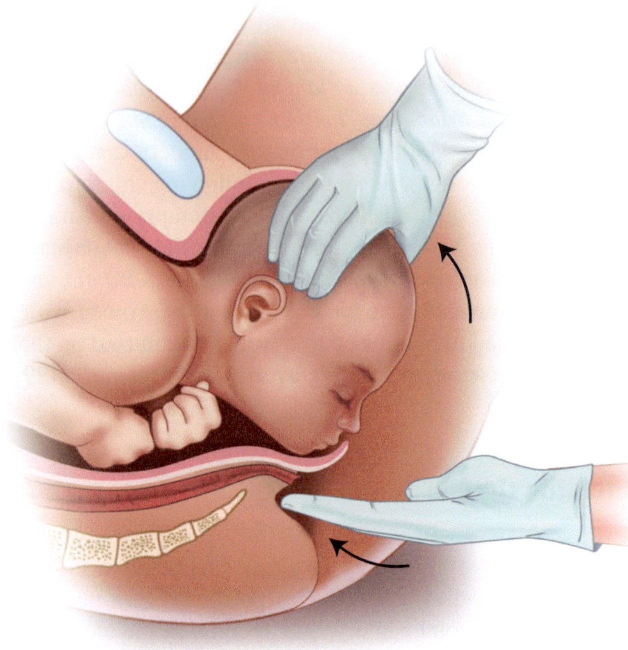

Fig. 1.1. Ritgen manoeuvre

p. 159). He instructed the pupil midwife to hold the fingers of her left hand, tips downward, over the vertex to prevent too rapid expulsion with the right hand supporting the perineum, with a clean pad covering the anus. He also described the practice of 'stripping' the perineum and 'chinning' the crowned head out which were similar to the Ritgen Manoeuvre.

During the twentieth century, most midwifery textbooks recommend some form of hand manoeuvres to protect the perineum during the second stage of labour, however due to lack of robust research evidence, most of the advice is based on the authors clinical experience, tradition or personal preference. Currently there remains lack of agreement regarding whether or not firm pressure should be applied to the fetal head to increase flexion, if the perineum should be supported and if the hands on versus the hands off or poised technique is more beneficial in preventing sever perineal trauma.

Methods Used to Restore Perineal Integrity

Sutures have been used to close wounds throughout the ages with 'eyed' needles being invented somewhere between 50,000 and 30,000 B.C. In 1600 BC the Edwin Smith papyrus shows that wounds were sewn with linen and silk thread. Other references indicate that linen strips coated with an adhesive mixture of honey and flour were used to close wounds similar to steri-strips. The writings of Hippocrates make reference to dry wounds healing well if the edges were kept closely approximated. Reference to catgut was made in 150 AD.

In the early seventeenth century needles were inserted into each side of the perineal wound and thread was wound over the needles to bring the skin edges together. This was similar to that used by East African tribes whereby they pushed Acacia thorns through the wound and then wrapped strips of vegetation around the protruding ends, in a figure of eight fashion, to close the trauma. Similarly porcupine quills were used.

In 1904, DeLee documented that it was customary to use silkworm gut to repair a '*perineorrhaphy*' or perineal laceration and stated that it '*may be boiled with the instruments unless already sterilized*' ([7], p. 117). He also described the removal of sutures from the perineum by the '*physician*' on the tenth day following delivery and stated that '*the patient should rest quietly for several hours after the sutures are removed*' ([7], p. 197).

During the early seventeenth century, Jacques Guillemeau [21] gave an account in his book entitled '*Childbirth or the Happy Deliverie of Women*' of how he successfully repaired the severely torn perineum of a woman who was 6 weeks post-delivery and "*both paffages (passages) were brought into one*" [21]. He described how he cut away the healed skin from each side of the wound and brought the edges together by winding thread over needles which had been inserted into each side of the perineum in a similar way that an '*harelip*' would have been repaired [21, 36].

In 1859, Doctor Mackesy from Waterford, Ireland gave an account of a woman who delivered her first child assisted by forceps. During the procedure she sustained damage to the perineum, which extended into the rectum. She was confined to bed for 3 weeks and made slow recovery but at 5 weeks postpartum she complained of faecal incontinence.

He went on to described how he repaired the trauma by cutting away the healed skin edges and inserting five interrupted iron wire sutures through the wound. The ends of the wires were passed through holes in two '*leaden plates*', which were placed each side of the wound. The wires were then tightened so that the edges of the wound were brought together with the strips of lead in close apposition and pressed down to the wound and the ends were then firmly secured with spilt lead shot [2] (Fig. 1.2).

The advantage of this method was that the wires could be tightened or loosened as required and could be left in place longer than silk or cord [5]. Black [4] also advised that in '*severe cases*' that the edges of perineal or vulval lacerations should be '*kept in contact by metallic sutures*'.

At the end of the nineteenth century Jellett [25] advised that lacerations of the perineum must be sutured immediately "*to avoid the formation of a puerperal ulcer and to guard against future prolapse of the uterus*". He recommended suturing the posterior vaginal wall separately with a continuous catgut suture and then repairing the perineal trauma with interrupted silkworm gut "*as it does not absorb the discharge*". The stitches were "*entered at the side of the laceration, passed completely beneath it, and brought out at the corresponding point upon the other side*" and then tied separately. However, Herman [23] stated that a "*few complete ruptures will heal without stitches and that it is difficult for an accoucheur single-handed to accu-*

Fig. 1.2. Repair of severe perineal trauma using wire sutures and lead strips

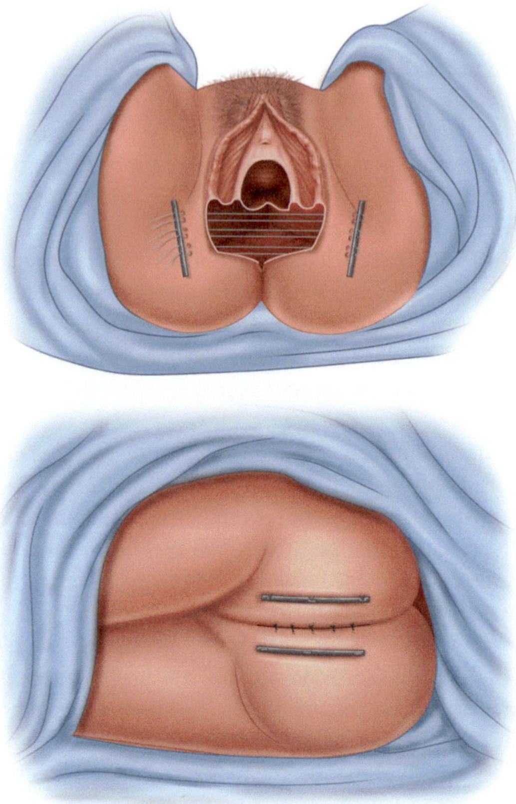

rately sew up an extensive rent". He also commented that "*if the perineum is badly stitched, the patient is no worse off than if it were not stitched at all; and if well stitched, the patient will be saved a great deal of future annoyance*".

Herman [23] advised that the repair should be performed under ether or chloroform anaesthetic, with the patient on her back with the "*thighs bent up and held apart so you may see its full extent*". In the late nineteenth and twentieth century catgut was used to repair tears because "*you have not the trouble of taking out the stitches but can leave them to be absorbed*" [23] whereas silkworm gut sutures usually had to be removed on the seventh day [25]. It was not until 1927 that local anaesthetic (novocaine) was introduced in obstetric practice by Gellhorn to ease the pain during delivery of the fetal head and prior to performing and suturing episiotomies [37].

It was many years before perineal suturing became generally accepted. This may have been due to the fact that insertion of stitches would have been extremely painful for women because there were no local anaesthetics. Moreover, equipment was very crude, aseptic techniques did not exist and most '*midwives*' were inexperienced in carrying out this procedure successfully.

In 1930 Rucker first reported using a continuous running stitch for repair of episiotomies or tears using silk-worm gut suture material to appose the deep tissues and superficial subcutaneous layer [38]. A continuous longitudinal mattress stitch was inserted to appose the vagina and 'levator fibres' and then a second row of sutures were inserted parallel to the first layer. Using this technique, the perineum was built up layer by layer with approximately four rows of sutures being inserted.

On completion of each layer the suture material was brought out through the skin to one side of the lower end of the wound and the upper ends of the four or five separate sutures were passed through a perforated shot and secured. Rucker reported that the patients were more comfortable following repair with this technique and the "results were uniformly excellent". The repair was completed by a continuous stitch to close the superficial submucous and subcutaneous tissues.

With the continuous suture technique there are no knots and "the sutures accommodate themselves to the swelling as it occurs", also there is no 'cutting' of the tissues by the stitches. He thought that it was difficult to know just exactly how tight or loose to tie interrupted sutures in order to allow for reactionary tissue swelling. Rucker postulated that if the sutures were tied too loosely then 'primary union' would not be achieved and if they were tied too tightly they were inclined to cut into the tissues and cause increased pain when swelling occurred.

Indeed, most women who had the 'Rucker' repair were unaware of having stitches and typically responded when questioned about perineal pain "Do I have stitches?" The operators found that this method was not technically difficult to perform and the additional few minutes spent on the repair was "more than justified by the gratitude of the mother because of the elimination or decrease in perineal pain".

In 1962 Christhilf and Monias tested a modified version of the 'Rucker' method in the USA on a series of 350 cases over a twenty-four month period. Assessment of this technique by Christhilf and Monias [6] was based purely on clinical impression and they made no attempt to repeat statistical evaluation of the procedure. Many of the patients were surprised that they had stitches and "contrasted the results favourably against previous experiences".

Christhilf and Monias [6] found that the continuous technique was rapid to perform, there were no significant infections, postpartum discomfort was minimal, healing was always by first intention and there were no wound breakdown or fistulae. Indeed, one wonders why the Rucker method never achieved more widespread knowledge or acceptance and why it was not described in textbooks. However, reference was made to a particular continuous suturing method that Chassar Moir evolved which was described in '*Munro Kerr's Operative Obstetrics*' textbook as being very similar to the method of repair described by 'Stuart and Monias' (1962) [31]. Note that the reference was incorrectly cited and that it should have been 'Christhilf and Monias' [6].

In 1990, Fleming published the findings from her experience of using a simple non-locking, continuous suturing technique for all layers, with subcutaneous stitches placed well below the perineal skin surface. Previous research highlighted the technical difficulty of carrying out subcuticular suturing but Fleming reported that the continuous method was easy to perform and could be easily taught to relatively inexperienced operators (N. Fleming, 1993, personal communication). She was taught this method by an obstetrician named William Schafer (her husband) with whom she worked in private practice.

The basic premise of this 'alternative' technique is that the sutures are placed 'loose and deep' in as few layers as possible in order to reduce the amount of foreign material implanted in the wound. The repair begins with an anchoring stitch above the apex of the vaginal trauma and the deep tissues and mucosa are closed with a single continuous 'running' stitch in comparison to the 'locking' stitch, which Christhilf and Monias used. Next the deep and superficial perineal muscles are re-approximated with a continuous, loose non-locking stitch with care taken to occlude the 'dead space'. The repair is completed with a continuous suture inserted well below the skin surface in the subcutaneous fascia to avoid the 'profusion of nerve endings' and is finished off with a terminal knot placed in the vagina. A single length of absorbable suture material is used for the repair with no knots other than the anchoring and terminal knot.

Fleming [14] reported that the "alternative repair technique results in a skin-edge gap of 2–3 mm" which initially caused some "personal uneasiness" regarding a possible increased risk of wound infection and the "long-term cosmetic results". The underlying principles of this 'alternative' loose continuous technique as described by Fleming [14] appear to be based on the method used by Christhilf and Monias [6]. However, Fleming was unaware of any of the previous work that had been carried out to evaluate continuous suturing techniques of perineal repair (N. Fleming, 2002, personal communication).

Fleming's doctorial research which was carried out in the suburban Chicago area, found surprisingly low levels of pain reported by women who were sutured with the loose continuous method "compared to general expectations and reports from other researchers" when more traditional suture methods were used. By 48 h postpartum the mean perceived perineal pain in both the laceration and episiotomy groups was rated as mild and by 2 weeks the women reported having virtually no pain [13]. At 6 weeks postpartum good cosmetic results were found on clinical examination and the scar was reported to be only of hairline thickness [14].

Fleming suggests that the suturing method may make a difference to the amount of postpartum perineal pain experienced by women. The 'alternative' continuous suturing technique used by Fleming appears to be associated with a lower incidence of pain compared with the results produced by other researchers using more traditional methods of perineal repair.

For more than 70 years researchers have been suggesting that continuous suture techniques of perineal repair are far better than interrupted methods in terms of reduced postpartum pain and yet they were not widely used until more recently [6, 10, 14, 20, 24, 28, 30, 33, 38]. Building on previous research, Kettle (2002) compared the loose non-locking continuous technique as described by Fleming [14] to the more traditional interrupted method of perineal repair. Results showed a significant reduction in perineal pain at 10 days postpartum compared to the traditional interrupted method.

Currently the continuous technique for repair of the vagina, perineal muscles and skin is widely used in the UK and internationally [26].

Training Issues

Throughout history midwifery is portrayed as being more of a social role with friends and neighbours being invited into the birthing chamber to help care for the woman during and after birth. Very few midwives could write about their experiences and therefore most skills relating to normal midwifery were passed down verbally from mother to daughter and they had no regulating body. During the sixteenth century women in the UK were formally licensed to practice 'midwifery' by the church and they received some instructions from '*men-midwives*' such as Willughby, Chamberlen and Smellie ([43], p. 55). However, midwives did not receive any formal training in the art and science of childbirth, until the late eighteenth century. In 1872 the London Obstetrical Society set up its own Board of Examiners and many thousands of midwives took an examination and successful candidates were issued with a certificate of competence to the ([36], p. 95). Following this, as a result of the 1902 Midwives Act, the Central Midwives Board (CMB) was established in England to regulate the training, supervision and registration of midwives.

Conclusion

In the twenty-first century the morbidity associated with perineal trauma remains an international issue with millions of women worldwide continuing to sustain some degree of perineal trauma following vaginal delivery. Implementation of standardised training programmes and evidence based practices may reduce the adverse sequalae of perineal trauma and make vaginal delivery more desirable. Practitioners who are appropriately trained are more likely to provide a consistent, high standard of perineal repair and hopefully will contribute to reducing the extent of morbidity and litigation associated with this procedure. Different approaches to teach these skills should be evaluated within the context of controlled trials.

References

1. Audit Commission. First class delivery: improving maternity services in England and Wales. London: Audit Commission Publications; 1997.
2. Beatty TE. Contributions to medicine and midwifery. Dublin: Fannin and Co.; 1866. p. 567.
3. Bender S. Obstetrics for pupil midwives. London: William Heinemann Medical Books Limited; 1968. p. 159.
4. Black JW. Selected obstetrical & gynaecological works of Sir James Y. Simpson, Bart. Edinburgh: Adam and Charles Black; 1871. p. 65.
5. Catalogue and report of obstetrical and other instruments. London: Longmans, Green and Co.; 1867. p. 172.

6. Christhilf SM, Monias MB. Knotless episiorrhaphy as a positive approach towards eliminating postpartum perineal distress. Am J Obstet Gynecol. 1962;84(6):812–8.
7. DeLee JB. Obstetrics for nurses. Philadelphia: W.B.Saunders; 1904.
8. DeLee JB. The prophylactic forceps operation. Am J Obstet Gynecol. 1920;1:34.
9. Derry DE. Note on five pelves of women of the Eleventh Dynasty in Egypt. J Obstet Gynaecol Br Emp. 1935;xiii:490–5.
10. Detlefsen GU, Vinther S, Larsen P, Schroeder E. Intradermal suturing of episiotomy wounds compared with interrupted sutures (transl). Ugeskr Laeger. 1980;142:3117–20.
11. Donald I. Practical obstetric problems. London: Lloyd-Luke; 1979.
12. Eccles A. Obstetrics and gynaecology in Tudor and Stuart England. 1st ed. London: Croom Helm Ltd; 1982.
13. Fleming N. Comparison of women with different perineal conditions after childbirth. Ann Arbor: UMI; 1987.
14. Fleming N. Can the suturing method make a difference in postpartum perineal pain? J Nurse-Midwifery. 1990;35(1):19–25.
15. Floud E. Protecting the perineum in childbirth 1: a retrospective view. Br J Midwifery. 1994;2(6):258–63.
16. Flood C. The real reason for performing episiotomies. World Med. 1982;17:51.
17. Gelis J. History of childbirth. 2nd ed. Cambridge: Polity Press; 1991.
18. Graham H. Eternal eve. Britain: William Heinemann Medical Books LTD; 1950.
19. Greenshields W, ulme H H. The perineum in childbirth: a survey of women's experiences and midwifery practices. London: National Childbirth Trust; 1993.
20. Guilhem P, Pontonnier A, Espagno G. Episiotomie prophylactique. Suture intradermique. Gynecol Obstet. 1960;59(2):261–7.
21. Guillemeau J. Child-birth or the happy deliverie of women. London: Printed by A Hatfield; 1612.
22. Harvie J. Practicle directions, shewing 'A Method of pefering the PERINǼUM IN BIRTH'. Printed for D. Wilson and G Nicol, London; 1767.
23. Herman GE. Difficult labour. A guide to its management for students and practitioners. London: Cassell and Company, Limited; 1898.
24. Isager-Sally L, Legarth J, Jacobsen B, Bostofte E. Episiotomy repair – immediate and long-term sequelae. A prospective randomized study of three different methods of repair. Br J Obstet Gynaecol. 1986;93:420–5.
25. Jellett H. A short practice of midwifery, embodying the treatment adopted in the Rotunda Hospital, Dublin. London: J & A Churchill; 1897. p. 282–36.
26. Kettle C, Hills RK, Jones P, Darby L, Gray R, Johanson R. Continuous versus interrupted perineal repair with standard or rapidly absorbed sutures after spontaneous vaginal birth: a randomised controlled trial. Lancet. 2002;359(9325):2217–23.
27. Kitzinger S, Walters R. Some women's experience of episiotomy. London: National Childbirth Trust; 1981.
28. Llewellyn-Jones JD. Commentary. Repair of episiotomies and perineal tears. Br J Obstet Gynaecol. 1987;94:92–3.
29. Magdi I. Obstetric injuries of the perineum. J Obstet Gynaecol Br Commonw. 1949;49:687–700.
30. Mandy TE, Christhilf SM, Mandy AJ, Siegel IA. Evaluation of the Rucker method of episiotomy repair as to perineal pain. Am J Surg. 1951;82:251–5.
31. Myerscough PR. Munro Kerr's operative obstetrics. 9th ed. London: Bailliére Tindall; 1977.
32. O'Dowd MJ, Philipp E. The history of obstetrics and gynecology. New York: The Parthenon Publishing Group; 2000.
33. Olah KS. Subcuticular perineal repair using a new continuous technique. Br J Midwifery. 1994;2(2):67–71.
34. Ould F. A treatise of midwifery. Dublin: Nelson and Connor; 1742.

35. Pomeroy RH. Shall we cut and reconstruct the perineum for every primipara? Am J Obstet Dis Woman Child. 1918;78:211–20.
36. Radcliffe W. Milestones in midwifery. Bristol: John Wright & Sons Ltd; 1967.
37. Rhodes P. A short history of clinical midwifery. 1st ed. Cheshire: Books for Midwives Press; 1995.
38. Rucker MP. Perineorraphy with longitudinal sutures. Virginia Med Mon. 1930;7:238–9.
39. Taliaferro RM. Rigidity of soft parts: delivery effected by incision in the perineum. Stethoscope Vaginia Med Gaz. 1852;2:383.
40. Temkin O. Soranus' gynaecology. Baltimore: The John Hopkins University Press; 1956.
41. Thacker SB, Banta HD. Benefits and risks of episiotomy: an interpretative review of the English language literature 1860–1980. Obstet Gynecol Surv. 1983;38(6):322–34.
42. Tew M. Safer childbirth? A critical history of maternity care. London: Chapman and Hall; 1990. p. 116.
43. Towler J, Bramall J. Midwives in history and society. Kent: Croom Helm Ltd; 1986.

Chapter 2
Anatomy and Physiology of the Pelvic Floor

Renaud de Tayrac, Katharina Jundt, Vincent Letouzey, Mélanie Cayrac, Florent Masia, Eve Mousty, Pierre Marès, Michel Prudhomme, Xavier Fritel, and Brigitte Fatton

Abstract The functional anatomy of the pelvic floor is based on a triple system of suspensor ligaments, cohesive fascia and muscle support. The integrity of these systems is essential if a normal anatomic and functional pelvi-perineal equilibrium is to be maintained. The levator ani is the principal muscle of the pelvic floor. It is made up mainly of the ileococcygeus muscle, that forms the levator plate, and the pubovisceral (or pubococcygeus) muscle which shares connective tract with adjacent organs and is divided into 2 bundles, the pubovaginal bundle and the puborectal bundle that is key to maintaining the pelvi-perineal functional equilibrium.

The pelvic floor plays many crucial roles in urinary continence, micturition, anal continence, defecation cycles, maintaining healthy sexuality and preserving the possibilities of pregnancy and normal childbirth. The fulfillment of all these roles depends on a complex and delicate balance that must be conserved.

The occurrence of pelvic floor disorders can be explained by successive exposures during life to congenital (tissue and anatomic factors), acquired (particularly obstetric trauma to the perineum), lifestyle and aging-related factors.

Adapted and translated from [1] Fatton B, Cayrac M, Letouzey V, Masia F, Mousty E, Marès P, Prudhomme M, de Tayrac R. Functional anatomy of the pelvic floor. Encyclopédie Médico-Chirurgicale. Gynecologie. Paris: Elsevier France; 2014.

R. de Tayrac (✉) • V. Letouzey • M. Cayrac • F. Masia • E. Mousty
P. Marès • M. Prudhomme • B. Fatton
Obstetrics and Gynecology Department, Caremeau University Hospital, Nimes, France
e-mail: renaud.detayrac@chu-nimes.fr

K. Jundt
LMU Munich/Frauenarztpraxis am Pasinger Bahnhof, August-Exter-Str. 4, 81245 Munich, Germany

X. Fritel
Obstetrics and Gynecology Department, Poitiers University Hospital, Poitiers, France

K.M.K. Ismail (ed.), *Perineal Trauma at Childbirth*,
DOI 10.1007/978-3-319-14860-1_2

Keywords Functional anatomy • Pelvic floor • Levator ani • Urethral sphincter • Anal sphincter • Genital prolapse • Cystocele • Uterus • Urinary incontinence • Fecal incontinence • Obstetric trauma

Descriptive Anatomy

Pelvic Muscles (*Fig. 2.1*)

The inner wall of the pelvis is lined with four muscle pairs surrounded by their fasciae: the piriformis muscle, the obturator internus muscle, the levator ani, and the coccygeal (coccygeus) muscle. The latter two muscles form the pelvic diaphragm which closes the lower pelvic outlet, separating the pelvic cavity from the perineum. The pelvic diaphragm has 2 hiatuses on its sagittal axis: anteriorly the urogenital hiatus containing the urethra and the vagina, and posteriorly the anal hiatus containing the anorectal junction.

The levator ani is the main muscle of the pelvic diaphragm, and consists of two parts:

- the static, posterolateral ileococcygeus muscle. This originates in the plane of the middle pelvic outlet at the posterior surface of the pubis, the tendinous arch of the levator ani and the inner surface of the ischial spine. It is a broad, thin muscle that passes downwards and backwards to terminate on the anococcygeal ligament and the lateral edges of the coccyx. It constitutes the "levator plate" which provides support for the pelvic organs during straining. This plate is more or less horizontal

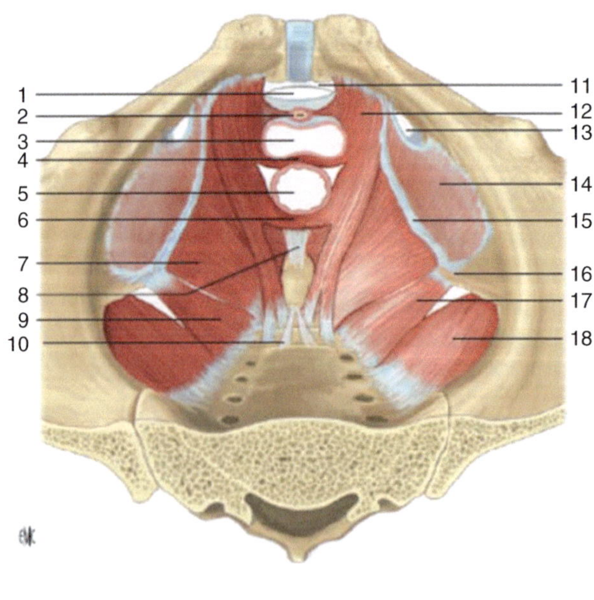

Fig. 2.1 Pelvic floor muscles. *1* Infrapubic hiatus; *2* urethra; *3* vagina; *4* pubovaginal muscle; *5* rectum; *6* puborectal bundle; *7* iliococcygeal muscle; *8* anococcygeal ligament; *9* coccygeal bundle; *10* ventral sacrococcygeal ligament; *11* arcuate ligament of the pubis; *12* pubococcygeus muscle; *13* obturator canal; *14* obturator muscle covered by its fascia; *15* Arcus tendineous levator ani; *16* ischial spine; *17* coccygeus muscle; *18* piriformis muscle (From Fatton et al. [1])

but moves vertically in cases of muscle weakening, causing a widening of the urogenital hiatus and thus promoting the occurrence of pelvic organ prolapse [2].

– the dynamic, anteromedial pubococcygeus muscle. This arises from the posterior surface of the pubis. It is a thick, powerful muscle that blends connective tracts with the fasciae of the viscera it encounters on its medial border, and hence also called the "pubo-visceral" muscle. It then splits into several bundles that terminate at the urethra, vagina, anus or rectum. These bundles can be clearly visualized by MRI but their description has led to considerable semantic confusion. Recently, based on MRI studies that precisely identified the points at which these bundles arise and terminate, it was suggested [3] that the pubovaginal, puboperineal, pubo-rectalis and puboanal would be suitable terms to describe the bundles that make up the puboviscenal muscle (term preferred over that of "pubococcygeus muscle" precisely because of these anatomical considerations).

From a functional point of view, three muscles have an essential role for the pelvic floor:

– the iliococcygeal muscle whose fibers make up the levator plate that provides support for the pelvic organs during straining.
– the pubovisceral muscle with its different components pubovaginal, puboperineal and puboanal.
– the puborectalis muscle whose contraction, by increasing the visceral caps, elevates the rectum, vagina and urethra. The puborectalis muscle is itself split into three bundles:

  • the lateralrectal bundle which terminates on the lateral wall of the rectum and whose fibers pass downwards to penetrate between the internal and external anal sphincters,
  • the retrorectal bundle that terminates on the anorectal angle,
  • the coccygeal bundle that terminates on the anterior surface of the coccyx and the ventral sacrococcygeal ligament.

The coccygeal muscle is an accessory muscle. It arises from the ischial spine, is triangular in shape, and is adherent to the sacrospinous ligament. It ends on the lateral edges of the coccyx and the lower sacrum (S4, S5).

It is also important to mention here that the levator ani muscle, like most postural muscles, is mainly made up of type I fibers [4]. Type I fibers are slow-twitch fibers that operate in oxidative mode and produce prolonged tonic contractions. This contrasts with type II fibers that operate primarily in anaerobic mode and whose contractions are rapid and fatigable. The upright posture particular to the human species compared to quadrupeds, and the consequent constant pressure exerted by the weight of the pelvic organs, could explain the high proportion of type I fibers in the levator ani muscle of humans. The proportion of type I fibers varies (66–90 %) depending on which fiber bundle in the levator ani muscle is considered, with the proportion of type II fibers increasing in the periurethral and perianal areas [4]. This suggests that the supporting muscles play a synergistic role: the permanent basal tone of the levator ani muscle can withstand the weight of the pelvic viscera in the upright posture, and the voluntary contraction of the pubovisceral bundle increases this tone when faced with a sudden increase in abdominal pressure [4].

The Perineum *(Fig. 2.2)*

The perineum constitutes all the soft tissue located below the pelvic diaphragm, closing the pelvic cavity. It is bounded anteriorly by the pubic symphysis, laterally by the ischio-pubic rami and the ischial tuberosities, and posteriorly by the apex of the coccyx. The perineum is divided into two triangular regions by an imaginary line connecting the ischial tuberosities: anteriorly the urogenital perineum, oriented downwards and forwards, and posteriorly the anal perineum, oriented downwards and backwards. The perineal body is located between these two perineal regions, on the midline and under the skin. This is a solid fibromuscular mass of imprecise boundaries. It is generally pyramidal in shape and forms an area onto which bundles of the pubovisceral muscle and perineal muscles are attached [5]. It is made up of elastin fibers, smooth muscle cells, and dense connective tissue.

The urogenital perineum is divided into two muscle layers: deep and superficial.

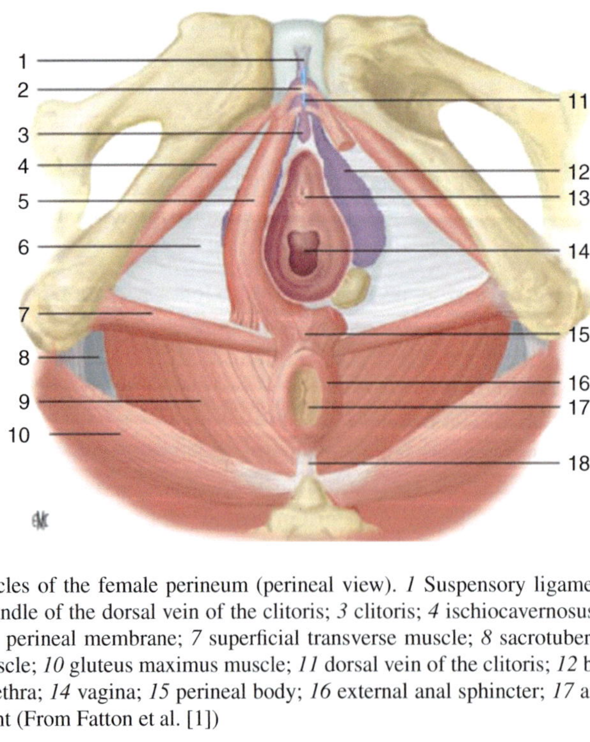

Fig. 2.2 Muscles of the female perineum (perineal view). *1* Suspensory ligament of clitoris; *2* compressor bundle of the dorsal vein of the clitoris; *3* clitoris; *4* ischiocavernosus muscle; *5* vestibular bulb; *6* perineal membrane; *7* superficial transverse muscle; *8* sacrotuberous ligament; *9* levator ani muscle; *10* gluteus maximus muscle; *11* dorsal vein of the clitoris; *12* bulbospongiosus muscle; *13* urethra; *14* vagina; *15* perineal body; *16* external anal sphincter; *17* anus; *18* anococcygeal ligament (From Fatton et al. [1])

- Superficial muscles of the urogenital perineum
  - The erector muscle: a muscle pair and close to the corpus cavernosum. It arises from the ischial rami, passes forwards and medially before terminating on the tunica albuginea of the corpus cavernosum. Its contraction compresses the corpus cavernosum.
  - The bulbospongiosus muscle: a muscle pair and close to the vestibular bulb. It arises from the perineal body, and passes forwards and medially. Along its path it covers the lateral side of the greater vestibular gland and the corresponding bulb, before terminating in the form of a posterior bundle on the body of the clitoris and an anterior bundle that merges above the deep dorsal vessels of the clitoris with its contralateral counterpart to form a strap. Its contraction compresses the dorsal vein of the clitoris, causing its erection, compresses the greater vestibular gland, and narrows the vaginal orifice.
  - The superficial transverse muscle of perineum: a thin and inconstant muscle pair. It originates from the inner surface of the ischial rami and terminates on the perineal body.
- The deep muscle of the urogenital perineum
  - The urethral sphincter muscle: surrounds the middle third of the urethra and is divided into two parts [6]:
  - The urethrovaginal muscle: circular fibers wrapped around the urethra and arcuate fibers attached frontally to the anterior and lateral sides of the vagina.
  - The compressor urethra muscle: transverse fibers stretched beneath the urethra and attached to the medial sides of the ischiopubic rami. Their possible bone attachments are still a matter of controversy, with favor currently being given to muscle attachments on the puborectalis bundle of the levator ani muscle [7].
  - The deep transverse muscle of perineum: a muscle pair of triangular shape. It originates from the inner surface of the ischial rami and terminates on the perineal body and vagina.

The anal perineum contains only one muscle: the external anal sphincter muscle. It encircles the lower part of the anal canal. It is divided into three parts, as follows from its surface to its depth: a subcutaneous portion forming a 15-mm flat plane, a superficial portion attached posteriorly to the ano-coccygeal ligament and anteriorly to the perineal body, and a deep, thicker portion which exchanges fibers with the puborectalis muscle (Fig. 2.3).

The Pudendal Nerve (Fig. 2.4)

Knowledge of its path and its many ramifications is essential to understand the painful perineal syndromes whose care is still today a challenge for the medical community.

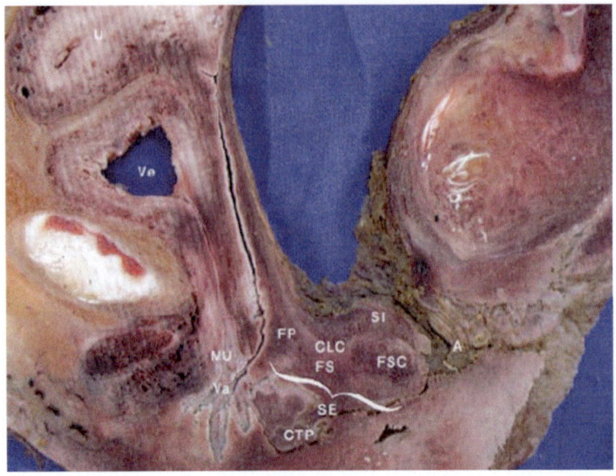

Fig. 2.3 Morphological anatomy of the anal sphincter. Sagittal section of a female pelvis through the sphincter. *A* anus, *CLC* complex longitudinal layer, *CTP* perineal body, *FP* deep bundle, *FS* superficial bundle, *FSC* subcutaneous bundle, *MU* urethral meatus, *SE* external sphincter, *SI* internal sphincter, *U* Uterus, *Va* vagina, *Ve* bladder

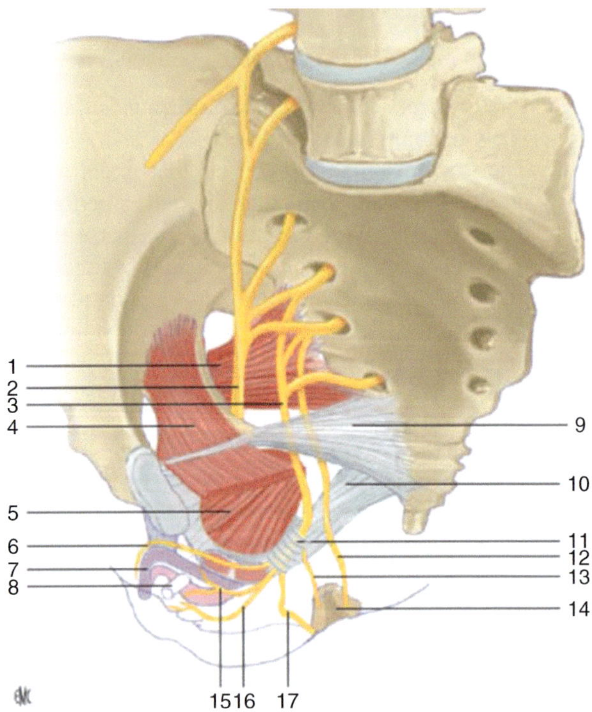

Fig. 2.4 Pudental nerve. *1* Piriformis muscle; *2* sciatic nerve; *3* pudental nerve; *4* sectioned levator ani muscle; *5* internal obturator muscle; *6* dorsal nerve of clitoris; *7* clitoris; *8* sectioned urethra; *9* sacrospinous ligament; *10* sacrotuberous ligament; *11* Alcock's canal; *12* superior rectal nerve; *13* medial rectal nerve; *14* external anal sphincter; *15* motor branch of the perineal nerve; *16* sensory branch of the perineal nerve; *17* inferior rectal nerve (From Fatton et al. [1])

The pudendal nerve originates in the pre-sacral region of sacral nerve roots S3, S4 and sometimes S2 [8], and is separate from the sciatic nerve that is lateral to it. It initially travels through the pelvic area in front of the piriformis muscle then through the greater sciatic opening before passing through the infra-piriformis foramen to the gluteal region. It travels a short distance here, behind the ischial spine or distal attachment point of the sacrospinous ligament. At this point it is located between the superior rectal nerve, medially, and the internal pudendal vessels, laterally. It crosses the lesser sciatic notch to join the ischio-rectal fossa, then travels through the pudendal canal described by Alcock that is formed by a splitting of the fascia of the obturator internus muscle. It is initially in the infra-levator position but becomes perineal as it travels along the ischio-pubic ramus in the deep perineal space. In Alcock's canal it gives rise to collateral branches such as the median rectal nerve and the perineal nerve which gives rise to the inferior rectal nerve (sensory nerve to the anal margin and the motor nerve of the external anal sphincter) then divides to form a superficial sensitive branch (sensory nerve to the labia majora) and a deep motor branch (deep transverse muscle of the perineum, bulbospongiosus muscle, erector muscle and striated urethral sphincter). The pudendal nerve ends as the dorsal nerve of the clitoris which travels above the transverse ligament of the perineum and passes through the pubic hiatus. It then intersects the lateral side of the suspensory ligament of the clitoris before following the back of the clitoris to the gland. Here it innervates the foreskin and the upper part of the labia minora.

The Normal Pelvi-Perineal Balance

The uniqueness and complexity of the pelvi-perineal balance reflects both the complementarity of muscle, ligament and fascial systems, and also their interdependence and synergy. This close relationship explains why a defect in one system may have effects and impacts on the others. Any damage to one system will overload and require adaptation by the other systems exposed. This organization that regulates pelvic stasis explains both the strength and the weakness of this balance. It needs to be fully understood if it is to be conserved or restored and it is this principle that should direct the teaching of pelvic perineology. This complementarity between the pelvic floor muscles, fascia and ligaments, which must be intact to maintain normal perineal stasis, is very well illustrated by the "boat in dry dock" image proposed by P. Norton [9]. If the muscle floor is deficient, the balance is maintained only by the fascial and ligamentous structures which are then subject to substantial forces. Any rupture or stretching of the ligaments, or any tearing of the fascia, will result in ptosis of the pelvic viscera. A biomechanical model has been used to illustrate more "scientifically" this interaction between muscle support and ligament suspension. Chen et al. [10] developed a model of the anterior vaginal wall and its various components of muscle and connective support (including the levator ani muscle, particularly its pubovisceral portion, uterosacral ligaments – cardinal ligaments complex). With this model they demonstrated that cystocele can be the result of altered muscle support, or damage to the ligament system, or a combination of the two. The role of the supporting muscle system is paramount. The greater the alteration in muscle support, the greater will be the anterior prolapse caused by damage to the ligament system. In a woman presenting with 60 % muscle damage, application in the model of 90 % damage to the uterosacral – cardinal ligament complex accentuated the anterior vaginal wall prolapse by 530 % (the lowest point sinking from 0.3 to 1.9 cm). An identical ligament injury, but in a woman presenting with 80 % muscle damage, accentuated the prolapse by 240 % (the lowest point sinking from 0.7 to 2.4 cm: it is here in this simulation that the largest cystocele was obtained). Conversely, if the floor muscle is normal, 90 % damage to the apical ligament does not induce any prolapse of the anterior vaginal wall.

The second step corresponds to the risk of perineal injuries that occur during pregnancy and childbirth. At expulsion, perineal stasis is modified by abdominal pushing and fetal descent. The puborectalis bundles of the levator ani muscle are driven apart, increase in length, then become superficial. Sphincter bundles are pushed laterally and backwards. Then, fetal presentation takes an oblique forward and upward direction. This causes distension of the perineum characterized by its thinning, an increase in anogenital distance, and vulvar distension. The perineal body becomes laminated, and from being triangular becomes curvilinear. These various modifications may cause muscle and/or aponeurotic and neurological injuries. Neurological damage, including stretching of the pudendal nerve (which will be discussed later), may be involved in the occurrence of prolapse, stress urinary incontinence and fecal incontinence.

Mechanisms of Urinary Continence and Urination

Appropriate continence and complete voiding of the bladder are absolute necessities for individuals to maintain healthy renal function and lead an active community life. This cycle is under voluntary control despite the fact that it is organized by means of reflex pathways.

Any factor that disturbs the balance of this cycle will induce pathologies that may have functional (incontinence, frequency) or physical (urolithiasis, infections, kidney failure) consequences.

Continence

Continence relies on the combined affect of several mechanisms.

1. ***Normal bladder compliance***: allows sufficient filling of the bladder while maintaining low intravesical pressure. Compliance is defined as the ratio of filling volume to intravesical pressure. It reflects the ability of the detrusor to allow itself to be distended, and therefore involves both the mechanical properties of the bladder and its innervation (autonomic nervous system) [11]. The sympathetic system allows the detrusor muscle to relax and inhibits its contraction.

   Compliance is investigated by means of urodynamic testing, primarily by cystometry. A study of bladder compliance throughout the filling phase showed that 75 % of this phase takes place at a pressure in excess of 10 ml/cm of H2O [12].

Compliance disorders are caused by alterations in bladder elasticity (for example in certain diseases such as radiation-induced cystitis, interstitial cystitis, bladder cancers, infectious disorders of the bladder, etc.). These bladder compliance disorders may also be caused by neurologic conditions (spinal cord injury, cauda equina syndrome, myelomeningocele, etc.).

In this context, reflex detrusor contractions and a lack of sphincter opening are often combined, causing high pressures in the bladder that are harmful for the upper urinary tract.

2. **Absence of bladder contractions during filling**: such contractions, if they occur, are the cause of the urgency, nocturia and frequency (that is sometimes precautionary), which characterize the clinical syndrome of an overactive bladder. Recent observations have established that this overactivity is not only related to an increase in detrusor contractility but also to an abnormality in the sensory processing that regulates continence [13]. This is supported by the fact that the urothelium is a highly specialized multimodal sensory organ that detects several physicochemical stimuli, transmits these stimuli to central structures, and communicates with adjacent structures (afferent nerves, smooth muscle fibers, myofibroblasts) causing their behavior to change. Any disruption of these functions will induce uncontrollable detrusor contractions.

   It is important here to distinguish between overactive bladder (OAB – clinical syndrome) and detrusor overactivity (urodynamic concept). Many studies have shown that OAB cannot be reliably detected by urodynamic testing: 60–80 % of symptomatic patients were undiagnosed by cystometry. In contrast, 10 % of detrusor contractions were seen to be uninhibited during recordings in healthy volunteers, and this figure even exceeded 40 % in ambulatory urodynamic testing [14]. Loss of bladder compliance and detrusor overactivity are the two mechanisms that cause urinary incontinence by OAB.
3. ***Role of bladder neck and urethra***: closure of the bladder neck and the smooth muscle urethral sphincter play a passive role in continence. In women, the urethra is approximately 40 mm long and 7 mm in diameter. It travels 30° from the vertical and, with the fundus of the bladder, forms the posterior urethrovesical angle. This angle is typically between 90° and 110°. A reduction or even the disappearance of this angle may be seen on relaxation of the supporting tissues. This phenomenon is involved in the mechanism of stress urinary incontinence in patients not suffering from sphincter deficiency.

For many years, the best test used to observe this angle was retrograde cystography with dynamic maneuvers, but this is performed only occasionally today in routine practice. It has been replaced by the simpler and safer perineal ultrasound scan that provides a reliable analysis of the cervico-urethral junction during rest and straining (see The Role of Imaging in assessing Perineal Trauma).

There are two layers of smooth muscle in the bladder neck and urethra:

- An inner layer of longitudinal fibers from the detrusor muscle, whose action is to open the bladder neck and shorten the urethra
- An outer layer consisting of circular, oblique fibers surrounding the bladder neck and the urethra. Conventionally, these fibers are considered to be a veritable

sphincter responsible for opening and closing the bladder neck and the urethra. But several observations suggest that they are not indispensable to the maintenance of continence: 20 % of young nulliparous women show stress opening of the bladder neck without incontinence [15]. Moreover, the zone of maximum urethral pressure lies in the middle third of the urethra, opposite the striated sphincter, not at the bladder neck.

It should also be noted that the submucosal vascular plexus is also to some extent involved in the continence mechanism.

Basal tone of the urethral striated sphincter, which acts as a security lock, is also involved in the continence mechanism [16]. This sphincter is composed of circular fibers and smooth muscle fibers. It extends over the entire length of the urethra but is circular only along its middle third. On the distal third, its fibers are attached to the lateral sides of the vagina (urethrovaginal muscle). It is reinforced at this point by the compressor urethra muscle (deep bundle of the bulbospongious muscle) made up of fibers stretched between the two ischiopubic branches and passing in front of the distal ureter. In 2003, Umek and DeLancey visualized these structures by MRI and measured the different segments of the urethra [17]: the segment surrounded by striated muscle starts 10–15 mm from the fundus of the bladder and extends over 20–35 mm.

Good quality urethral support (Fig. 2.5). The distal vagina, which makes up DeLancey's level III [18], is in direct and intimate contact with neighboring structures (urethra, levator ani muscle in their paramedian portion). The urethra is maintained here by connective tissue support reinforced by muscle/fascia connections.

This description constitutes the theory of the suburethral hammock and is far removed from the concept of Enhorning manometric assessment. Ulmsten and Petros [19] proposed a comprehensive theory in which they combined the suburethral hammock with the pubourethral ligaments that are actively involved in maintaining continence.

These similar, complementary theories led to the development of sub-urethral tapes (urethral stabilization techniques) that over the last decade have completely

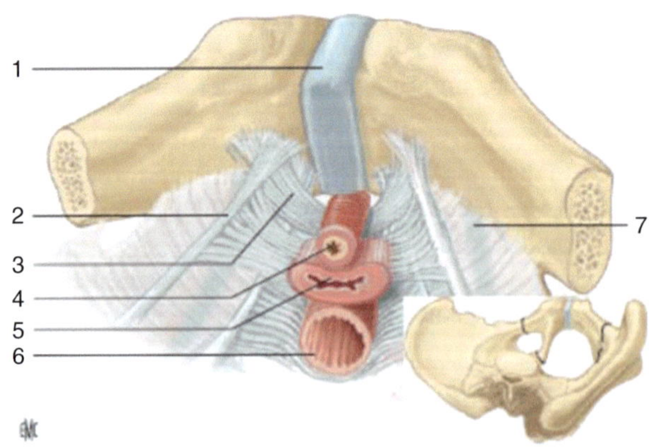

Fig. 2.5 Urethral support (Adapted from DeLancey JO, Am J Obstet Gynecol 1994). *1* Pubic symphysis; *2* arcus tendineous fascia pelvis (ATFP); *3* fascial and muscle connections; *4* urethra; *5* bladder; *6* rectum; *7* pelvic diaphragm (From Fatton et al. [1])

replaced the traditional Burch colposuspension operation [20] in the treatment of stress urinary incontinence (SUI) in women. Thus, the pathophysiological mechanisms involved in SUI in women are hypermobility of the cervico-urethral axis (not defective support structures) and sphincteric deficiency (not damage to the urethral sphincter), and these two mechanisms may sometimes be combined. Effective management of this incontinence should therefore be based on a rigorous analysis of the mechanisms involved: the hypermobility may be diagnosed clinically whereas sphincteric deficiency, if it has a clinical expression, is an urodynamic concept.

Micturition

In adults, micturition is under voluntary control involving striated muscle, but it also brings the autonomic nervous system and smooth muscle fibres into play. The mechansm must ensure rapid and complete bladder emptying, and this requires both contraction of the detrusor and relaxation of the different urethral sphincters. These two mechanisms are dependent upon somatic and vegetative innervations.

Detrusor muscle: this forms an expandable pouch composed of smooth muscle fibers and is fixed on a rigid bladder base rich in connective tissue where the ureters and urethra enter the bladder. Conventionally, the detrusor wall is considered to consist of a triple cell layer, but in fact it is more of a plexiform structure in which the individual fibers are intertwined [21]. This constitution explains the formation of muscle spans or even diverticula in cases of high-pressure voiding (obstruction, bladder sphincter dyssynergia).

The bladder and urethra are supplied with triple innervation:

- Parasympathetic (cholinergic) innervation that is dominant and responsible for motor control of the detrusor muscle. The nerve fibers originate from the sacral center (S2–S4). They follow the path of the pelvic splanchnic nerves and form the inferior hypogastric plexus.
- Sympathetic (adrenergic) innervation. Its nerve endings are more numerous at the bladder fundus. It contributes to maintaining the tone of the smooth muscle fibers in the internal sphincter and thus to bladder relaxation. The nerve fibers originate from the lumbar dorsal center (T10-L1). They follow the path of the splanchnic nerves, along the lateral side of the aorta, and form the superior hypogastric plexus. This gives rise, on either side, to the hypogastric nerves that join the inferior hypogastric plexus.
- Non adrenergic and non cholinergic (NANC) innervation: This plays a complex role, with ubiquitous sites of action (central and/or peripheral nervous system) and may act directly (peptide neurotransmitters) and/or indirectly (neuromodulation, cotransmission) [22].

It is therefore easy to understand that any injury to the pelvic splanchnic nerves or inferior hypogastric plexus will result in voiding dysfunction through urinary retention.

Voluntary (somatic) innervation of the urethral sphincter striated muscle**:** its center is in Onuf's nucleus located in the ventral part of the anterior horn of the spinal cord, from S2 to S4. Its nerve fibers form the motor part of the pudendal nerve. This innervation allows voluntary contraction of the sphincter striated muscle and of the different pelvic floor muscles.

Somatic and sympathetic activity causes inhibition of the parasympathetic system and ensures that the detrusor muscle does not contract during filling.

Mechanisms of Anal Continence and Defecation

This is governed by an equally complex balance. Maintaining anal continence is an essential requisite for an active social life. It is acquired in infancy and involves a set of organs and anatomical structures that are dependent upon both the voluntary and autonomic nervous systems. Continence can only be maintained and defecation can only be exerted if the relevant anatomical structures are intact and an appropriate balance is established between the two nervous systems.

Continence

Continence is ensured by a reservoir, the descending colon, and the sigmoid colon that is extended by the rectum, which is closed by a twin sphincter system (Fig. 2.3). The levator ani muscle, and more particularly its puborectalis bundle, also plays a role in maintaining anal continence.

Rectum: This is located at the lower part of the gastrointestinal tract and is 12–15 cm long. It extends from the rectosigmoid junction (at S3) to the anal orifice. The lower half of the rectum is located below the peritoneum.

A distinction is made between the pelvic rectum and the perineal rectum (or anal canal).

– Pelvic rectum: Viewed from the front, the pelvic rectum bends in the form of an "S" in italics, with two bends to the right (upper and lower) and one to the left (middle). These bends form grooves (externally) and Houston's valves (internally). The largest volume in the rectal reservoir is located in the lower part of the pelvic rectum (rectal ampulla). At the rectosigmoid junction, colonic bands turn into a longitudinal muscle layer that is more extensive on the anterior and posterior surfaces than on the sides. The walls of the rectum have viscoelastic properties that allow low-pressure filling (in the same manner as in the bladder) [23]. At the pelvic diaphragm (levator ani muscle), the pelvic rectum bends backwards, forming the anorectal flexure, and becomes the perineal rectum. The anorectal angle is 90° at rest. Maintenance of this angle plays an important role in anal continence. Normally, the rectum is empty. The rectosigmoidal junction protects the rectum by obstructing peristaltic waves [24]. This mechanism only works for solid stool and may be overwhelmed during episodes of diarrhea.

- Perineal rectum (or anal canal): This is on average 4 cm long. It extends during voluntary retention and shorten during defecation. Its mucous membrane lining is separated into two parts by the pectinate line. The upper half of the lining forms a series of longitudinal reliefs (Morgagni columns) which are joined at their base by mucosal folds known as anal valves. Anal glands open into the canal at this point and lubricate fecal material passing through. The mucosa is of the colorectal type and covers the hemorrhoidal arteriovenous internal plexus. A gray-blue, very fine, non-keratinized, hair- and gland-free squamous epithelium is located beneath the pectinate line extending to the edge of the anus.

The anal sphincter (Fig. 2.6): This plays a major role in maintaining anal continence. It is in fact made up of two circular sphincters: the internal sphincter and the external sphincter.

These are separated by longitudinal fibers, forming the longitudinal muscle of the anus.

- The internal sphincter: This consists of a circular arrangement of smooth muscle fibers and is a continuation of the rectal muscularis of which it constitutes a thickening. These fibers are whitish and distinct from the red fibers of the striated sphincter. It is between 0.5 and 4 mm thick. Endoanal ultrasound scan shows this as a very hypoechoic, circular structure of consistent thickness (See chapter on Imaging).
- The external sphincter: This consists of striated muscle fibers, but its anatomic description remains controversial [25]. It may be made up of one, two or three bundles, depending on the author. The fibers of which it is constituted appear to be intertwined with different bundles of the levator ani muscle. MRI has shown the anal sphincter to be a ring involving the outermost part of the sphincter, with the deepest part being formed by the puborectalis bundle of the levator ani muscle.

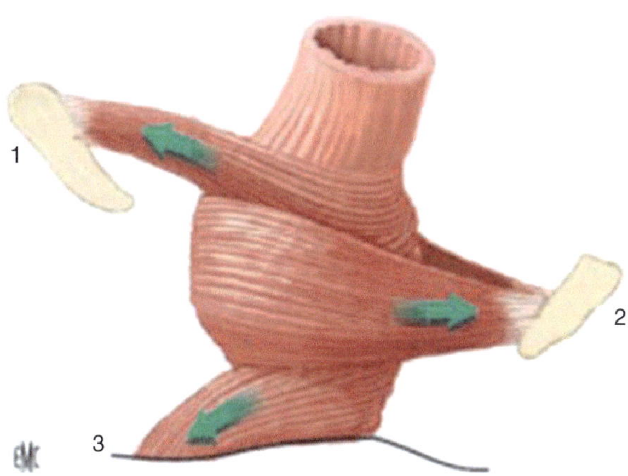

Fig. 2.6 Triple-loop organization of the external anal sphincter (Adapted from Shafik A, Invest Urol 1975). The top loop is formed by the puborectal strap *1* which is attached to the pubis, passes behind the lower rectum and maintains an angle of about 90° between the rectum and the anus. The intermediate loop of the external anal sphincter *2* is anchored to the coccyx. The base loop of the external anal sphincter *3* is attached to perianal skin (From Fatton et al. [1])

Shafik put forward a model that has the advantage of taking account of the sphincter's anatomic and functional synergy, and includes a description in the form of a triple-loop system [26] (Fig. 2.6):

- A base loop that is attached frontally to perianal skin and passes beneath the anal canal beyond the internal sphincter. It forms the edge of the external orifice of the anal canal.
- An intermediate loop that originates on the dorsal side of the coccyx and passes in front of the anal canal. It constitutes the superficial bundle of the external sphincter.
- A top loop formed by the puborectalis bundle of the levator ani muscle constituting the deep bundle of the external anal sphincter. It originates from the pubis and passes behind the anal canal. The puborectalis muscle therefore plays a fundamental role: since it is wrapped around the anorectal junction, its basal tone maintains the anorectal flexure and explains the radiological footprint on the posterior wall of the rectum that is visible on defecography images.

These three loops contract in opposite directions and thereby close the anal canal.

The longitudinal anal muscle*:* this forms a fibrous muscular sleeve located in the intersphincteric space. It is made up of fibers from the pelvic parietal fascia, smooth muscle fibers from the rectal muscularis, and striated muscle fibers from the levator ani muscle. Its contraction causes a shortening of the anal canal and promotes defecation.

The mechanism of continence: At rest, the autonomous, continuous contraction of the internal anal sphincter creates an area of high pressure (5–9 kPa) in the anal canal. As intrarectal pressure at rest does not exceed 1 kPa, no leakage of gas or stool is possible. This tone of the internal sphincter muscle is of myogenic origin but is also dependent upon extrinsic innervation of the sphincter since damage to the hypogastric nerves or sacral nerve roots is detrimental to this tone. Conversely, it is not diminished by complete spinal cord injury. Its maintenance is therefore autonomous in the spinal cord.

Should intra-abdominal pressure suddenly rise (e.g., during laughing, coughing, physical exercise), intrarectal pressure exceeds 20 kPa and therefore threatens anal continence. A reflex contraction of the external anal sphincter may be observed in these situations. This reflex is preserved in spinal patients. It is not under voluntary control. The magnitude of the sphincter contraction is directly correlated to the intra-abdominal pressure.

The arrival of air or feces in the rectum causes [25]:

- Rectal contraction (rectorectal reflex)
- Relaxation of the internal sphincter (rectoanal inhibitory reflex)
- Contraction of the external sphincter (rectoanal excitory reflex)

This sequence of stereotyped events constitutes the anorectal sampling reflex since relaxation of the internal sphincter brings rectal contents into contact with the upper part of the anal canal where specialized receptors determine the different characteristics of the fecal bolus (gas, liquid, solid). Contraction of the external sphincter protects continence during this analysis. Any disorder of anorectal sensitivity (neurological disease, surgical trauma) may disrupt this analysis and cause fecal incontinence.

Should immediate defecation be impossible (which is generally the case), rectal compliance will ensure that the bowel movement is deferred. Rectal distension induces a sensation of need, which is directly correlated to the tension exerted on the rectal walls. This sensation is processed in the cortex, and whereas it is initially transient for small filling volumes, it becomes permanent and ultimately intolerable.

Defecation

The aim of defecation is to achieve complete rectal emptying, under voluntary control. It involves several phenomena, both reflex and voluntary. The initiation of rectal emptying is controlled by the cerebral cortex.

The different steps to achieve defecation are as follows:

- Anorectal sampling reflex without contraction of the external sphincter, i.e. contraction of the lower part of the colon associated with relaxation of the internal sphincter. This contraction has the capacity to empty the entire left colon.
- Relaxation of the puborectalis sling associated with a lowering of the pelvic floor which narrows the anorectal angle. A defect in this relaxation, called anorectal asynchrony, induces terminal constipation or dyschezia. This condition is evidenced in defecography by the persistence of a large anorectal angle during defecation, associated with incomplete rectal emptying.

Afferent innervation from the different effector organs ends in nerve centers located in the cerebral cortex, amygdala, midbrain and medulla. The cortex plays a key role in coordinating, and particularly inhibiting, rectal emptying. However, a complete defecation reflex is possible in cases of complete spinal cord injury, triggered by perineal stimulation. A spinal center is therefore capable of coordinating the various mechanisms involved in defecation.

During normal defecation, relaxation of the puborectalis muscle opens the anorectal angle, causes the rectum to become vertical, and lowers the pelvic floor. The sphincters relax, and this gradually opens and shortens the anal canal. The propulsive force induced by the rise in intrarectal pressure has two sources: firstly contraction of the rectal ampulla associated with closure of the rectosigmoid junction, and secondly contraction of the diaphragm and abdominal muscles during straining [27].

Pelvi-Perineal Anatomy and Pregnancy and Childbirth

Pregnancy

Although obstetric trauma is one of the causes of pelvic floor disorders, pregnancy itself is also known to have an effect (due to high abdominal pressure and associated hormonal changes) which explains why prophylactic cesarean section does not completely protect the pelvic floor.

The anatomical changes that occur in the lower urinary tract during pregnancy mainly affect the bladder. It is pushed forward and upward by the gravid uterus. The trigone, which is normally concave, becomes convex, and in particular alters the orientation and position of the ureteral meatus. The lateral stretching of the ureters shortens their path beneath the mucosa, exposing them to vesicoureteral reflux.

Pregnancy is accompanied by enhanced connective tissue laxity, lumbar hyperlordosis, mobility of the sacroiliac joints and relaxation of the abdominal muscles. This in addition to the forward movement of the uterus, as it increases in size, leads changes the direction of pressure from the anococcygeal region to the urogenital hiatus. These changes may have a direct clinical impact on the pelvic floor, with pregnant nulliparous women showing a higher pelvic organ prolapse score than non-pregnant nulliparous women: a case-control study involving 21 women evaluated during their first pregnancy found POPQ stage 2 prolapse in 47.6 % of cases, while all the women in the control group showed POPQ stage 0 or 1 [28]. Additionally, ultrasound scans have confirmed this specific effect of pregnancy with early ptosis of the bladder neck at rest: this deficiency in urethral support may persist to a lesser extent after childbirth [29, 30].

Childbirth and Obstetric Trauma

A close link (relative risk of four to ten) has been established between vaginal delivery and the risk of prolapse [31], although the level of evidence is still low. At childbirth, the neuro-muscular damage that occurs – in addition to the morphological changes to the bladder and pelvis/perineum – constitutes a risk factor for prolapse and urinary and fecal incontinence [32].

However, although prolapse and urinary and/or fecal incontinence have been shown in short- and medium-term studies to be more common after vaginal delivery than after cesarean section, these differences are less obvious at the long-term [33]. In addition, no significant difference was noted when the strength of the pelvic floor muscles is compared after cesarean section and vaginal delivery [34]. Finally, the anatomic changes and symptoms observed after a first childbirth are not or only slightly modified by subsequent deliveries [35].

Other factors such as age, estrogen levels, genetic factors and overweightness play a role in the pathophysiology of pelvic floor disorders [33]. The bony anatomy of the pelvis, as mentioned above, could also be involved in prolapse. However, MRI pelvimetry cannot reliably pinpoint patients at risk. Significant association is found between fecal incontinence and a markedly concave sacrum [36].

Morphological changes: the changes undergone by the urethra and bladder during childbirth are morphologically well known; during engagement, the urethra is flattened against the symphysis pubis and the bladder neck is pushed upward and forward [1]. The perineum undergoes different anatomical changes at the different stages of childbirth [27]. After engagement in one of the diameters of the pelvic inlet, the fetus begins its descent into the pelvic cavity: the pelvi-coccygeal bundle of the levator ani muscle causes flexion and rotation of the fetus, then distends in order to open the urogenital slit. Pressure from the fetus causes retropulsion of the coccyx which results in stretching of the posterior commissure of the anus. Thus, in the initial stages of engagement, it is the posterior perineum that is the first to be called upon and distended. During maternal pushing, the puborectalis bundle also contracts and this raises the perineal body, draws the anal canal upward, and dilates the anus [27]. It is only later, on deflexion of the fetal head, that the anterior perineum is distended. The puborectalis bundle is pushed downward and forward, the perineal body stretches, ano-vulval distance lengthens to double its normal length (from 3–4 to 12–15 cm), and the vulvar orifice enlarges. Crossing the incision in the levator ani muscle is the key timeline in freeing the head of the fetus [37]. The superficial perineum is then the last obstacle to fetal expulsion. The vulvar ring becomes horizontal and expands until it reaches the size of the large circumference of the fetal head.Childbirth, and particularly expulsion, can thus cause injuries to the perineum, especially to its muscles. The risk of tearing the puborectalis bundle at its anchor point on the perineal body is all the greater if the diameter required to free the fetus is large (occipito-posterior presentation exposes the perineum to more injury than occipito-pubic presentation.

After delivery, urethral mobility is increased by Valsalva maneuver. This increase does not take place after caesarean section but is maximal after using forceps or a vacuum.

Muscle damage: damage to the puborectalis muscle is a common feature of vaginal delivery and appears as more or less extensive visible "defects" by ultrasound scan [38] or MRI. The risk of such lesions occurring is increased after a forceps delivery (OR 3.4) [39]. Damage such as this enlarges the muscle hiatus [40] and increases the risk of genital prolapse. These lesions of the levator ani muscle and their relationship with prolapse were described for the first time in 1907.

Currently, an odds ratio of 5.7 has been calculated between lesions of the levator ani muscle and prolapse, but this may be underestimated [41].

The levator ani muscle, and especially its puborectalis bundle, is of particular functional importance as it is involved in the continence mechanisms and contributes by its basal tone to maintaining the anatomo-functional balance. This muscle, however, is exposed to substantial stress during childbirth as it needs to stretch to three times its usual length [42]. This distension enlarges the hiatus of the levator ani muscle and allows passage of the fetal head. Ultrasound scans before and after childbirth have confirmed that the hiatus is enlarged postpartum, suggesting that passage of the fetal head is the main risk factor for damage to the levator ani muscle [43]. This hypothesis is supported by the fact that no damage is found after cesarean section [44].

The prevalence of levator ani lesions is between 15 and 30 % in women who undergo vaginal delivery. Today, this prevalence is increasing as the probability of muscle damage may increase with maternal age at first birth [41].

The use of birth instruments poses the greatest risk. Forceps increase the frequency of levator ani muscle injury with an odds ratio of between 3.83 and 10.47 [44]. A large head circumference (>35.5 cm) and long second stage of labor

(>110 min) could be other independent risk factors [45]. Epidural analgesia would appear to have a protective effect.

This damage to the levator ani muscle during childbirth is often caused by what Dietz called "levator avulsion" whereby the muscle is detached from its anchorage on the lower branch of the pubis and the tendinous arch of the levator ani muscle [46]. The lesion is located at the bone/muscle interface, and is not therefore a lesion of the muscle itself. It results in a para-rectal retraction of the muscle. Most of these lesions are located on the right side, but may also be bilateral [47]. They are diagnosable at childbirth if combined with vaginal damage, but in most cases are hidden and are therefore difficult to diagnose clinically. The development of imaging techniques, first MRI then 3D ultrasound, has rendered the diagnosis of these lesions more accurate and more reliable.

In addition to providing a direct visualization of muscle avulsion, imaging can also measure muscle hiatus (transverse diameter or area) and distances been the muscle attachment point and the urethra or symphysis.

The hiatus increases substantially in size immediately following vaginal delivery compared to cesarean delivery. This increase is thought to be correlated with the circumference of the fetal head [48]. Also, it has been shown that the hiatus is significantly greater in area in women presenting with genital prolapse [49].

Avulsion of the levator ani muscle could be one of the missing links between vaginal delivery and the development of pelvic organ prolapse. Several studies have established a correlation between genital prolapse and injuries of the levator ani muscle. Women presenting with avulsion of the levator ani muscle had twice the risk of developing grade 2 or higher prolapse [42]. The association was strongest for uterine prolapse (RR = 4.0) and cystocele (RR = 2.3) [42]. Efforts should therefore be made in the future to detect risk factors such as muscle damage in order to propose rules for primary prevention. Likewise, the pertinence of repair surgery should be questioned in efforts to reduce the risk of subsequent prolapse in the women concerned.

Neurological and neuromuscular injuries: as well as damaging muscles – sometimes without any apparent skin lesions – childbirth may also have a neurological impact: stretch neuropathy and neurogenic damage to the perineal muscles or sphincter. All these are risk factors for prolapse and/or urinary and/or fecal incontinence. Childbirth, and particularly the expulsion phase, may cause partially reversible perineal denervation affecting the nerve structures of the pelvic organs and muscle floor. These neurological lesions are associated with muscle deficiency which can be documented by manometric measurements [50]. In this matter, the pudendal nerve and its branches have been the subject of most studies. A long expulsion phase, a forceps delivery or a high birth weight are significantly associated with an increase in pudendal nerve latency. Caesarean section is protective if elective. Recovery would appear to occur over the first 3 months after childbirth, with signs of reinnervation on electromyographic recordings, and lesion stability thereafter [51]. Uncertainties remain regarding the precise role of delivery method and the length of the expulsion phase which may be decisive.

Many studies have been conducted on pelvic floor muscle strength before and after childbirth, using either palpation or a vaginal manometer. They showed a

25–35 % decrease in the muscle strength of the pelvic floor post partum [51]. This decrease would appear to be temporary and in most cases resolves within 1 year [52]. This muscle damage would appear to be less marked following caesarean section [53].

Damage to the anal sphincter: women who undergo vaginal delivery have a relative risk of two to three of subsequently suffering fecal incontinence as this form of delivery is the main etiology of anal sphincter injuries [54]. The increasingly widespread use of endoanal or postnatal perineal ultrasound techniques has helped determine that the prevalence of anal sphincter injuries, particularly occult forms [55], is high. Typical risk factors include nulliparity, posterior presentations, instrumental delivery, fetal macrosomia, and poor control during freeing of the fetal head. Anal sphincter injuries are associated with an increased risk of medium- or long-term fecal incontinence [56]. However, most anal sphincter lesions are occult and are detectable only by ultrasound scan. In this case they are usually asymptomatic [35] but may be a risk factor for the development of secondary fecal incontinence, particularly during menopause.

Pelvi-Perineal Anatomy and Sexuality

Human sexuality is managed by a very complex alchemy that cannot be restricted to simple anatomical considerations, far from it. Nevertheless, the role of the levator ani muscle during intercourse is important both in terms of the biology of reproduction and the quality of the coitus for both the woman and her partner [1].

A number of studies have sought to clarify objectively the role of the levator ani muscles in coitus and sexual performance. Shafik [57] talks of the "vagino-levator reflex". In 17 women he studied the electromyographic response of the levator ani muscles to vaginal distension achieved by inflating a condom with 300 ml of air: the amplitude and duration of the activity recorded increased with vaginal distension. He also noted that this response became exhausted after several successive distensions, probably due to muscle fatigue. Thus, during intercourse, vaginal distension by the erect penis causes contraction of the levator ani muscle which induces vaginal narrowing and elongation, and this provides appropriate "congruence" with the penis that increases in rigidity. In addition, under the combined effect of the contraction of the sphincter portion of the levator ani muscle, and of the puborectalis and pubovaginal bundles, the uterus moves upward and the top third of the vagina swells to create a better receptacle for sperm, thus optimizing the conditions for reproduction.

An approach based on an anatomical and dynamic description of coitus with vaginal penetration during MRI is most appealing given the quality and comprehensiveness of the analysis it provides. However, it is limited by the number of possible positions and the difficulties inherent to recording certain sequences. An initial study recorded face-to-face intercourse using the T2 sequence on the sagittal plane. In this position, before penetration, the vagina was seen to be parallel to the pubococcygeal axis with moderate anterior convexity. After penetration, this convexity was accentuated by the glans penis which pushed against the anterior fornix of the vagina. The posterior wall of the bladder was pushed upwards and forwards, and the uterus was pushed upwards and backwards [58]. A second experiment was conducted with MRI images in all three planes during intercourse to ejaculation in the "doggy style" or "super G" position. In th position the penis pushed against the posterior fornix, and the bladder and the uterus were pushed forwards [59]. Each position corresponds to a specific contact area, stimulation of specific areas, the displacement of pelvic organs, and the tensioning of certain ligaments. Thus, MRI may help to better assess the synergies and other anatomic "connections" involved during intercourse [59].

From a purely anatomical point of view, MRI can be used to determine which organs are displaced and are therefore involved in sexual intercourse. Contrast agents may also be injected to investigate changes in vascularization during sexual intercourse, particularly during arousal. MRI analysis with gadolinium in post- and premenopausal women showed that the vestibular bulb and the width of the labia minora increased with arousal. No changes in the labia majora, urethra, cervix or rectum were observed during sexual arousal. MRI is thus able to provide information on the functional changes that occur during the different stages of sexual intercourse [60].

Several studies have shown that there is no correlation between the size of the vagina and the quality of vaginal sex. Shortening the length of the vagina (except in extreme cases) is not associated with the onset of sexual dysfunction [61, 62].

A prospective cohort study in heterosexual women aged over 40 years showed that the size of the vagina correlated with sexual activity (9.1 ± 1.2 cm versus 8.9 ± 1.3 cm in non-sexually active women, $p = 0.04$), but this correlation disappeared after adjustment for age. The total length of the vagina and size of the vaginal orifice did not differ in women with a normal Female Sexual Function Index (FSFI) score and those with a sexual dysfunction [63].

The famous "G spot" is still the subject of debate, with opinions hesitating between its consideration as a true anatomical entity and a mental representation of the area that is the very embodiment of female pleasure. A recent literature review provided an overview of this topic that is still controversial and concluded on the need for more scientific studies. It would appear that the location of the G spot on the anterior vaginal wall is anatomically variable from one woman to another [64].

Our knowledge of the physiology of female sexuality and of the mechanisms involved in the disorders thereof is fragmentary, but the (particularly functional) contribution made by MRI should provide a better understanding of the complex connections that govern sexuality in women.

Conclusion

Although knowledge of fundamental descriptive anatomy is essential to our understanding of the female perineum, dynamic functional anatomy adds another dimension and creates a crucial link between physiology and pathophysiology. Anatomy comes "alive" and the pelvic floor is no longer a simple inert platform but a veritable dynamic diaphragm with many important functions. Modern imaging techniques and the development of ever more accurate anatomic models have meant that pelvic floor disorders can now be better diagnosed. It is this better understanding of functional anatomy that will allow us to optimize primary means of prevention which may preserve the perineum throughout life despite traumatic events such as pregnancy and above all childbirth.

References

1. Fatton B, Cayrac M, Letouzey V, Masia F, Mousty E, Marès P, Prudhomme M, de Tayrac R. [Functional anatomy of the pelvic floor]. Encyclopédie Médico-Chirurgicale. Paris: Elsevier France; 2014 .p. -. French.
2. Hsu Y, Summers A, Hussain HK, Guire KE, Delancey JO. Levator plate angle in women with pelvic organ prolapse compared to women with normal support using dynamic MR imaging. Am J Obstet Gynecol. 2006;194:1427–33.
3. Margulies RU, Huebner M, DeLancey JO. Origin and insertion points involved in levator ani muscle defects. Am J Obstet Gynecol. 2007;196:251.e1–5.
4. Yiou R, Costa P, Haab F, Delmas V. Functional anatomy of the pelvic floor. Prog Urol. 2009;19:916–25. French.
5. Larson KA, Yousuf A, Lewicky-Gaupp C, Fenner DE, DeLancey JO. Perineal body anatomy in living women: 3-dimensional analysis using thin-slice magnetic resonance imaging. Am J Obstet Gynecol. 2010;203:494.e15–21.
6. Rahn DD, Roshanravan SM. Pathophysiology of urinary incontinence, voiding dysfunction, and overactive bladder. Obstet Gynecol Clin N Am. 2009;36:463–74.
7. Wallner C, Dabhoiwala NF, DeRuiter MC, Lamers WH. The anatomical components of urinary continence. Eur Urol. 2009;55:932–43.
8. Robert R, Prat-Pradal D, Labat JJ, et al. Anatomic basis of chronic perineal pain: role of the pudendal nerve. Surg Radiol Anat. 1998;20:93–8.
9. Norton PA. Pelvic floor disorders: the role of fascia and ligaments. Clin Obstet Gynecol. 1993;36:926–38.
10. Chen L, Ashton-Miller JA, Hsu Y, Delancey JO. Interaction among apical support, levator ani impairment, and anterior vaginal wall prolapse. Obstet Gynecol. 2006;108:324–32.
11. Chartier-Kastler E, Ayoub N, Even-Schneider A, Richard F, Soler JM, Denys P. Neurogenic bladder: pathophysiology of abnormal compliance. Prog Urol. 2004;14:472–8. French.
12. Gilmour RF, Churchill BM, Steckler RE, Houle AM, Khoury AE, McLorie GA. A new technique for dynamic analysis of bladder compliance. J Urol. 1993;150:1200–3.
13. Kerdraon J, Siproudhis L. Pathophysiology of overactive bladder. Lett Med Phys Readapt. 2010;26:69–73. French.
14. Digesu GA, Khullar V, Cardozo L, Salvatore S. Overactive bladder symptoms: do we need urodynamics? Neurourol Urodyn. 2003;22:105–8.
15. Chapple CR, Helm CW, Blease S, Milroy EJ, Rickards D, Osborne JL. Asymptomatic bladder neck incompetence in nulliparous females. Br J Urol. 1989;64:357–9.
16. Mauroy B, Bonnal JL. Anatomo-radiological basis of urinary incontinence. In: Es LC, editor. Urinary and fecal incontinence. Multidisciplinary approach. Ipsen Biotech, Beaufour Ipsen, Dreux, France; 2001. p. 1–19. French.
17. Umek WH, Kearney R, Morgan DM, Ashton-Miller JA, DeLancey JO. The axial location of structural regions in the urethra: a magnetic resonance study in nulliparous women. Obstet Gynecol. 2003;102:1039–45.

18. DeLancey JO. Structural support of the urethra as it relates to stress urinary incontinence: the hammock hypothesis. Am J Obstet Gynecol. 1994;170:1713–20. discussion 1720–3.
19. Petros PE, Ulmsten UI. An integral theory of female urinary incontinence. Experimental and clinical considerations. Acta Obstet Gynecol Scand Suppl. 1990;153:7–31.
20. Paraiso MF, Walters MD, Karram MM, Barber MD. Laparoscopic Burch colposuspension versus tension-free vaginal tape: a randomized trial. Obstet Gynecol. 2004;104:1249–58.
21. Hunter DTJ. A new concept of urinary bladder musculature. J Urol. 1954;71:695–704.
22. Buzelin JM, Labat JJ. Physiologie de la continence urinaire et anale. Pelvi-périnéologie. 2005;31–44.
23. Moore KL, Dalley AF. Anatomie Médicale: aspects fondamentaux et applications cliniques. Bruxelles: De Boeck et Larcier; 2007. p. 395.
24. Baker WNW, Mann CV. The rectosigmoid junction zone: another sphincter ? In: Thomas PA, Mann CV, editors. Alimentary sphincters and their disorders. London: MacMillan Publishers LTD; 1981.
25. Leroi AM. Anatomy and physiology on anal sphincter. In: Amarenco G, Chantraine A, editors. Sphincter function. Paris: Springer, France; 2006. p. 27–49 .French.
26. Shafik A. A new concept of the anatomy of the anal sphincter mechanism and the physiology of defecation. The external anal sphincter: a triple-loop system. Investig Urol. 1975;12:412–9.
27. Villet R, Buzelin JM, Lazorthes F. Female pelvi-perineal disorders. Paris: Vigot; 1995 .French.
28. O'Boyle AL, Woodman PJ, O'Boyle JD, Davis GD, Swift SE. Pelvic organ support in nulliparous pregnant and nonpregnant women: a case control study. Am J Obstet Gynecol. 2002;187:99–102.
29. Peschers U, Schaer G, Anthuber C, Delancey JO, Schuessler B. Changes in vesical neck mobility following vaginal delivery. Obstet Gynecol. 1996;88:1001–6.
30. Yang JM. Factors affecting urethrocystographic parameters in urinary continent women. J Clin Ultrasound. 1996;24:249–55.
31. Mant J, Painter R, Vessey M. Epidemiology of genital prolapse: observations from the Oxford Family Planning Association Study. Br J Obstet Gynaecol. 1997;104:579–85.
32. Fatton B, Jacquetin B. Pelvic and perineal sequelae of delivery. Rev Prat. 1999;49:160–6. French.
33. Aukee P, Tihtonen K. Pregnancy, delivery and pelvic floor disorders. Duodecim. 2010;126:2381–6.
34. Baytur YB, Serter S, Tarhan S, Uyar Y, Inceboz U, Pabuscu Y. Pelvic floor function and anatomy after childbirth. J Reprod Med. 2007;52:604–10.
35. Jundt K, Scheer I, Schiessl B, Karl K, Friese K, Peschers UM. Incontinence, bladder neck mobility, and sphincter ruptures in primiparous women. Eur J Med Res. 2010;15:246–52.
36. Handa VL, Lockhart ME, Kenton KS, et al. Magnetic resonance assessment of pelvic anatomy and pelvic floor disorders after childbirth. Int Urogynecol J Pelvic Floor Dysfunct. 2009;20:133–9.
37. Merger R, Levy J, Melchior J. [Normal delivery]. Obstetrics. Paris: Masson; 1985. p. 115–36. French.
38. Eisenberg VH, Chantarasorn V, Shek KL, Dietz HP. Does levator ani injury affect cystocele type? Ultrasound Obstet Gynecol. 2010;36:618–23.
39. DeLancey JO, Miller JM, Kearney R, et al. Vaginal birth and de novo stress incontinence: relative contributions of urethral dysfunction and mobility. Obstet Gynecol. 2007;110:354–62.
40. Ismail SI, Shek KL, Dietz HP. Unilateral coronal diameters of the levator hiatus: baseline data for the automated detection of avulsion of the levator ani muscle. Ultrasound Obstet Gynecol. 2010;36:375–8.
41. Dietz HP. Levator trauma in labor: a challenge for obstetricians, surgeons and sonologists. Ultrasound Obstet Gynecol. 2007;29:368–71.
42. Dietz HP, Simpson JM. Levator trauma is associated with pelvic organ prolapse. BJOG. 2008;115:979–84.

43. Blasi I, Fuchs I, D'Amico R, et al. Intrapartum translabial three-dimensional ultrasound visualization of levator trauma. Ultrasound Obstet Gynecol. 2011;37:88–92.
44. Cassado Garriga J, Pessarrodona Isern A, Espuna Pons M, et al. Four-dimensional sonographic evaluation of avulsion of the levator ani according to delivery mode. Ultrasound Obstet Gynecol. 2011;38(6):701–6.
45. Valsky DV, Lipschuetz M, Bord A, et al. Fetal head circumference and length of second stage of labor are risk factors for levator ani muscle injury, diagnosed by 3-dimensional transperineal ultrasound in primiparous women. Am J Obstet Gynecol. 2009;201:91.e1–7.
46. Kim J, Ramanah R, DeLancey JO, Ashton-Miller JA. On the anatomy and histology of the pubovisceral muscle enthesis in women. Neurourol Urodyn. 2011;30:1366–70.
47. Dietz HP. Quantification of major morphological abnormalities of the levator ani. Ultrasound Obstet Gynecol. 2007;29:329–34.
48. Falkert A, Endress E, Weigl M, Seelbach-Gobel B. Three-dimensional ultrasound of the pelvic floor 2 days after first delivery: influence of constitutional and obstetric factors. Ultrasound Obstet Gynecol. 2010;35:583–8.
49. DeLancey JO, Morgan DM, Fenner DE, et al. Comparison of levator ani muscle defects and function in women with and without pelvic organ prolapse. Obstet Gynecol. 2007;109:295–302.
50. Allen RE, Hosker GL, Smith AR, Warrell DW. Pelvic floor damage and childbirth: a neurophysiological study. Br J Obstet Gynaecol. 1990;97:770–9.
51. Dietz HP, Wilson PD. Childbirth and pelvic floor trauma. Best Pract Res Clin Obstet Gynaecol. 2005;19:913–24.
52. Elenskaia K, Thakar R, Sultan AH, Scheer I, Beggs A. The effect of pregnancy and childbirth on pelvic floor muscle function. Int Urogynecol J. 2011;22:1421–7.
53. Sigurdardottir T, Steingrimsdottir T, Arnason A, Bo K. Pelvic floor muscle function before and after first childbirth. Int Urogynecol J. 2011;22:1497–503.
54. Meyer S, Achtari C. Female anal sphincter pathology during pregnancy and childbith. In: Amarenco G, Chantraine A, editors. Sphincter function. Paris: Springer; 2006. p. 195–229. French.
55. Fatton B, Jacquetin B. [Micturition disorders during pregnany and delivery]. Female urinary incontinence. Paris: Elsevier; 1998. p. 21–87. French.
56. Wegnelius G, Hammarstrom M. Complete rupture of anal sphincter in primiparas: long-term effects and subsequent delivery. Acta Obstet Gynecol Scand. 2010;90(3):258–63.
57. Shafik A. The role of the levator ani muscle in evacuation, sexual performance and pelvic floor disorders. Int Urogynecol J Pelvic Floor Dysfunct. 2000;11:361–76.
58. Faix A, Lapray JF, Courtieu C, Maubon A, Lanfrey K. Magnetic resonance imaging of sexual intercourse: initial experience. J Sex Marital Ther. 2001;27:475–82.
59. Faix A, Lapray JF, Callede O, Maubon A, Lanfrey K. Magnetic resonance imaging (MRI) of sexual intercourse: second experience in missionary position and initial experience in posterior position. J Sex Marital Ther. 2002;28(Suppl 1):63–76.
60. Suh DD, Yang CC, Cao Y, Heiman JR, Garland PA, Maravilla KR. MRI of female genital and pelvic organs during sexual arousal. J Psychosom Obstet Gynaecol. 2004;25:153–62.
61. Given FTJ, Muhlendorf IK, Browning GM. Vaginal length and sexual function after colpopexy for complete uterovaginal eversion. Am J Obstet Gynecol. 1993;169:284–7. discussion 287–8.
62. Weber AM, Walters MD, Piedmonte MR. Sexual function and vaginal anatomy in women before and after surgery for pelvic organ prolapse and urinary incontinence. Am J Obstet Gynecol. 2000;182:1610–5.
63. Schimpf MO, Harvie HS, Omotosho TB, et al. Does vaginal size impact sexual activity and function? Int Urogynecol J. 2010;21:447–52.
64. Jannini EA, Whipple B, Kingsberg SA, Buisson O, Foldes P, Vardi Y. Who's afraid of the G-spot? J Sex Med. 2010;7:25–34.

Chapter 3
Perineal Mapping

Vladimir Kalis, Magdalena Jansova, and Zdenek Rusavy

Abstract Perineal mapping is the complex analysis of the impact of anatomical conditions and interventions during the final phase of vaginal birth on risk of maternal perineal trauma. It includes tests on physical or computational models, experimental measurements on human tissues or clinical evaluation of different factors at the time of birth.

Experimental perineal mapping utilises data obtained from different sources such as stereophotogrammetry, virtual simulations, direct physical measurements and ultrasonography or other imaging techniques. Clinical perineal mapping involves data analysis based on the size of the fetal head, length/diameter of the genital hiatus, dimensions and elasticity of the perineal tissues or the co-operation of the parturient. This allows for individualised selection of certain modifications from a set of obstetric interventions e.g. use of obstetric gel, type and timing of episiotomy, manual perineal protection, slowing of the passage of the fetal head, second stage perineal massage, local application of warm packs. These interventions are employed to decrease frictional forces, increase the diameter of the vaginal introitus, decrease the size of the passing object, disperse/decrease the perineal tension, increase the elasticity of the perineum and/or control the speed of the delivery of the fetus and to harmonize all complex processes with the maternal efforts.

With the use of perineal mapping, an international classification of episiotomies has been developed and the effectiveness of manual perineal protection has been evaluated based on biomechanical principles while considering a variety of its modifications. Other interventions are in line for future analysis.

V. Kalis, MD, PhD (✉) • Z. Rusavy, MD, PhD
Department of Gynecology and Obstetrics, Biomedical Center, Faculty of Medicine, Charles University and University Hospital Pilsen, Pilsen, Czech Republic
e-mail: KALISV@fnplzen.cz

M. Jansova, PhD
New Technologies – Research Centre, University of West Bohemia, Pilsen, Czech Republic

K.M.K. Ismail (ed.), *Perineal Trauma at Childbirth*,
DOI 10.1007/978-3-319-14860-1_3

Keywords Perineal trauma • Definition • Classification • Perineal mapping • Obstetric intervention • Manual perineal protection • Episiotomy

Introduction

In spite of case reports of occult anal sphincter injury diagnosed after caesarean section with no previous vaginal delivery [12], the main cause of perineal injury is at the time of vaginal birth.

Recent studies have evaluated maternal characteristics and obstetric variables and consequently identified risk factors for perineal trauma. Some of these factors have been widely acknowledged while others were found disputable and were not fully agreed upon (see Chap. 4). However, commonly, the accepted risk factors (vaginal nulliparity, fetal macrosomia and occipito-posterior position) are mostly non-modifiable and their mere identification is not helpful in reducing the rate and/or degree of perineal trauma in routine obstetric practice.

Furthermore, a number of events and obstetric interventions occurring at the end of the second stage of labour, when perineal structures are at the highest risk of tearing, have not been rigorously evaluated (Table 3.1) due to technical or ethical difficulties to achieve the evidence. Globally, we strive for "evidence-based practice" and hence, in the context of peri-partum interventions there is tendency to ignore interventions that lack such strong evidence base [25, 64, 74, 75]. Nevertheless, these interventions are commonly employed in clinical obstetrics [1, 19, 34, 50–53, 78, 79]. The complex analysis of the effect of maternal and fetal anatomical conditions and obstetric interventions utilisable during the final phase of vaginal birth on the risk of maternal perineal trauma is termed perineal mapping.

There are two types of perineal mapping, experimental and clinical. **Experimental perineal mapping** consists of a set of tests made on birthing models or experimental measurements on parturient women using the principles of biomechanics. **Clinical perineal mapping** consists of fast data collection and evaluation made in routine clinical practice at the time when the fetal head crowns the perineum.

Experimental Perineal Mapping

To date, experimental perineal mapping has been used less commonly compared to clinical perineal mapping. The most commonly used technique has been virtual perineal mapping (see sections "Virtual Perineal Mapping" and "Perineal Mapping and the Biomechanics of the Manual Perineal Protection During the Expulsion of the Fetal Head").

Table 3.1 Interventions and their variations considered for use during the final phase of vaginal delivery

Intention	Cogitable intervention	Variable applicable/assessability
Decrease in frictional forces	Obstetric gel	
Increase in the diameter of the vaginal introitus	Episiotomy	Type (location) of episiotomy Timing Length
Decrease in the size of the passing object	Manual perineal protection (MPP) during the expulsion of the fetal head	Flexion/extension of the fetal head by the anterior hand of the accoucheur
	MPP during the delivery of the shoulders	Extension of the fetal head by the posterior hand of the accoucheur Approximation of the posterior shoulder to the pubic bone Delivery of the posterior shoulder prior to the anterior shoulder
Redistribution of the perineal tension	MPP during the expulsion of the fetal head	Type of MPP
	MPP during the delivery of the shoulders	Type of MPP
Increase in the elasticity of the perineum	Slowing of the passage of the fetal head	Controlling the speed of expulsion of the fetal head by the anterior hand of the accoucheur Maternal co-operation: minimisation of pushing during expulsion
	Perineal massage Warm packs on the perineum Waterbirth	Perineal massage during the 2nd stage
Acceleration of the delivery of the fetus	Instrumental delivery	Forceps Vacuum extraction Thierry's spatula
	Episiotomy	Type of episiotomy Timing of episiotomy
	Fundal pressure – Kristeller's maneuver	By palm By forearm
Complex understanding and use of all suitable steps	Individuality of the obstetrician/midwife	Dexterity
	Individuality of the parturient	Experience Education Maternal co-operation: pushing when expected
Avoidance of fetal passage through the perineum	2nd stage caesarean	

Stereophotogrammetry

As the deformation in the perineal region during a vaginal birth occurs in three dimensions, it is not possible to capture this from one single angle or position. Stereophotogrammetry is a non-invasive method that allows for the analysis of deformations in three-dimensional space.

It works on a similar principle to human vision. An object in space is photographed from two different positions at the same time [86] (Fig. 3.1). In order to know the exact position of the object in space using the referential system, the scene must be calibrated first by taking a pair of images from a calibration grid and calculating the coordinates in the reference system of the chosen points on that grid. For calibration, it is necessary to know the location and orientation of the cameras along with the parameters of their lenses.

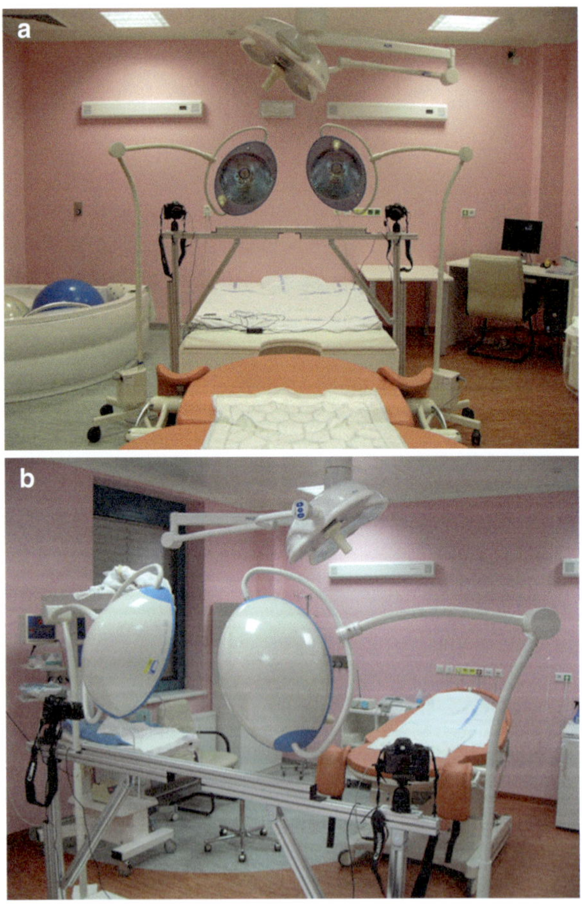

Fig. 3.1 (**a**, **b**) Stereophotogrammetry setting

When the object is photographed, its surface can be reconstructed from given points/marks on the object. Hence, comparing its state before and after change can assess its deformation.

In case of the perineum, the perineal skin can be marked with distinctly colored dots, such as brilliant green, gentian violet or site skin markers. The points visible in each time frame during vaginal delivery are used to create a mesh composed of surface elements (see Fig. 3.2). The coordinates of every point are calculated for each time frame. Subsequently the strains (deformations) are calculated for each element. A deformation field is determined on the mesh representing the visible surface of the perineum during a vaginal birth.

Application of Stereophotogrammetry in Clinical Practice

The results of a study using stereophotogrammetry have shown that the maximum tissue strain is located at the posterior fourchette [86]. This maximum strain is mainly orientated transversely. The transverse strain has been found to be more than four times higher than the maximum antero-posterior strain [86]. Considering this, interventions that reduce or disperse the maximum tissue tension at the fourchette may be beneficial in reducing the rate and degree of perineal trauma.

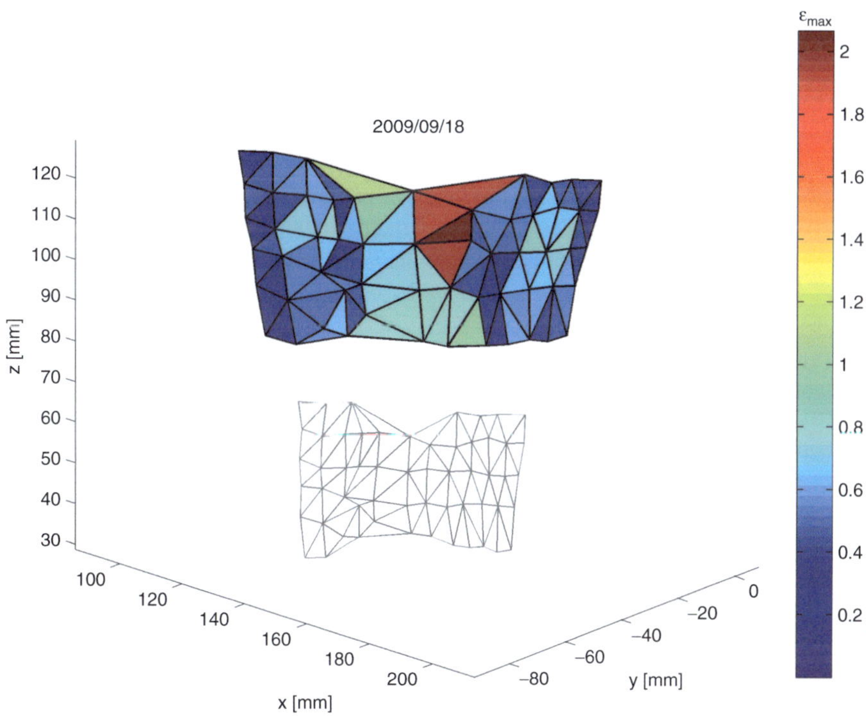

Fig. 3.2 Stereophotogrammetric mesh composed of surface elements

Virtual Perineal Mapping

In order to predict the behavior of tissue under load, it is possible to create a virtual (computational) model. Such analysis of the behaviour of tissues under load was made possible thanks to the progress in computing in recent decades. One approach is based on a finite element method [87]. The principle lies in an object being divided into elements interconnected by nodes, fixed in space and loaded corresponding to a given reality. Each element is then represented by a set of differential equations. These equations are solved to obtain an approximate solution describing the state of each element at a given time. To design this model, the initial geometry of the female pelvic floor at the beginning of the second stage of labour is based on available data from previous experimental, clinical and biomechanical studies.

The following anatomical, mechanical and clinical parameters should be chosen to define the biomechanical model to improve how accurately it corresponds to the dynamic changes in perineal anatomy during the final stage of labour:

1. Perineal parameters
   (a) The location and dimensions (length, thickness, angle) of the perineal structures (e.g. symphysis pubis, subpubic angle, inferior pubic rami, genital hiatus, perineal body, anus),
2. Fetal parameters
   (a) Fetal head dimensions,
   (b) Trajectory of the passage of the fetal head,
3. The accoucheur's parameters
   (a) Location of the thumb and the index-finger on the perineal surface,
   (b) Area of contact between fingers and the perineum,
   (c) Coordinated movement between fingers and its vector.
4. Tissue parameters
   (a) Mechanical properties
5. Boundary conditions
   (a) Motion constraints

Developing the Model of the Perineum (Fig. 3.3)

The model geometry and the surface mesh of the perineum and surrounding tissue can be created either from available image data (e.g. MRI data) using a specialised software, e.g. open source Slicer, or commercial Amira® (FEI Visualization Sciences Group, Burlington, MA, USA) or Simpleware ScanIP (Simpleware Ltd., Exeter, UK) or from scratch based solely on known dimensions using pre-processor software, e.g. HyperMesh (Altair, Troy, MI, USA), Catia (3DS, Vélizy-Villacoublay, FR).

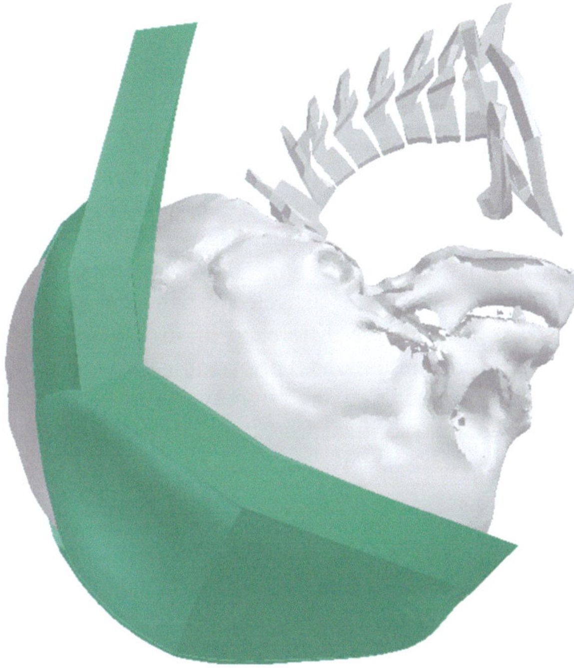

Fig. 3.3 Virtual model of the perineum and fetal head

Elastic, viscoelastic or hyperelastic material models are usually used for soft biological tissues [28]. Because the perineal tissue undergoes extensive deformation during vaginal delivery [86], an elastic material model is not suitable. From the point of view of finite element modeling, vaginal delivery is a long and slow process that can be performed by quasi-static simulation. For viscoelastic material, long–time simulations are required to properly assess the viscosity of the perineal structures because the loading response of viscoelastic material depends on the strain rate and the loading history. However, simulation of the second stage of vaginal delivery, which is considered a long process as it lasts several minutes, with the aid of viscoelastic material would require excessive computational cost. In contrast, a hyperelastic material model is suitable for large deformations and its response is not dependent on the strain rate, which allows for a shortening of the simulation without compromising the correct material response. Therefore, hyperelastic material seems to be suitable for this study at the present time [36, 37, 55].

In general, when modeling living tissues, there is a problem in obtaining data describing the tissue behaviour under load. In case of perineal tissue due to the lack of such data, the material parameters can be selected after repeated simulation tests and evaluations can be performed based on their realistic behaviour during the simulation. The shape of the bulging of the perineum and the previous experimental data (e.g. the dilation of the vaginal introitus, or the change in the perineal body length) serve for this evaluation. It is imperative before running any simulation studies that the model is validated, i.e. checked if its behaviour corresponds to reality. In an ideal case, it means running a simulation corresponding to an experiment with given boundary conditions. The model of the perineum is then validated for realistic bulging of the perineum [37].

In order to prepare the model for simulation, the boundary conditions are applied. The soft tissue has to be fixed in space with respect to the anatomy. The tissue connection of the inner area behind pubic rami to the bone is simulated by fixed displacements. The outer edge of the model is fixed for all degrees of freedom. At present, the absolute values of stress cannot be compared to other studies due to differences in selected material parameters, but it is possible to compare the relative difference in stress/tension between particular versions of the model simulations. For example the peak of stress in the hands-off simulation was selected as the reference value of 100 % and the results of simulations of manual perineal protection (MPP) were related to its value as percentages [36, 37].

Developing the Model of the Fetal Head (Fig. 3.3)

For the development of the numerical model of the realistic moulded fetal head either MR, CT or 3D laser scan images of the full-term neonatal skull or existing skull models can be used. Depending on the model requirements it is not always necessary to account for details like fossae, foramina and sulci. To save computational time, the fetal head can be modeled as a rigid body, i.e. an object that cannot be deformed. The trajectory of the fetal head can be set so that it moves as close as possible to the pubic rami, which simulates the movement of the fetal head along the curve of Carus during vaginal delivery.

Advantages

The main advantage of virtual perineal mapping is that it follows correct methodological criteria enabling the evaluation of the impact of vaginal birth and peripartum conditions on the perineum based on robust biomechanical principles. Furthermore, virtual models enable evaluation of a variety of modifications of a single intervention (e.g. various types of MPP), while all other variables and conditions remain unchanged (i.e. constant birthing conditions where only the analysed variable is changed). Obviously, this is not feasible in real clinical settings. Similarly, one can assess the impact of a fixed intervention on different maternal and fetal conditions (e.g. different fetal head size, positions or perineal dimensions). A major benefit of virtual mapping is that simulation can be stopped at any given time (e.g. expulsion of the fetal head) and hence, the timing of the measurement is very precise, such precision would not be possible in a clinical setting.

Finally, one major advantage is that with technological advances models are constantly improving allowing the generation of refined data without the ethical challenges of real life measurements.

Current Limitations

The main limitation of most models incorporating human body tissues is the lack of data regarding the material parameters, in this case it is the perineal tissue. Ideally, material parameters would be obtained from experimental measurements. However, this is difficult for many reasons: Firstly, the ethical considerations of obtaining tissue samples for this purpose; Secondly, tissue samples are usually taken from elderly and non-pregnant donors and therefore may have different material properties and thirdly, tissues behave differently "in vivo" compared to "in vitro".

In general, finite element models are, to some degree, usually a simplification of reality. This simplification occurs at different levels – omitting tissues, which are not expected to affect the results, simplifying the shape of tissue or tissue constraints and by using homogenous instead of heterogenous material. With regards to perineal models for vaginal delivery, the following simplifications are possible; omitting levator ani, simplification of the shape of the perineum on the cross section, the use of a premoulded fetal head, imposing fetal head trajectory directly instead of modeling the pushing effort.

As the tissue response to loading can only be analysed at the level of elements and their nodes, it is not possible to obtain detailed information at the level of muscle cells.

Application of Virtual Perineal Mapping in Clinical Practice

So far the computational perineal mapping has been used to evaluate MPP during the expulsion of the fetal head (see Sect. 3.3.2).

Direct Measurement on the Perineum

A direct measurement on the perineum can replace the more sophisticated stereophotogrammetry. The advantage here is that this measurement is not affected by the position of the accoucheur in front of the camera to avoid the head or shoulder getting in the way of the light.

A correct methodological approach is essential regarding the precision of the markings on the perineum along with the measurement and timing of the process. The same markers discussed in section "Stereophotogrammetry" can be used for drawing the lines or dots. This method has been used by several authors for measurements of episiotomy characteristics (e.g. the distance from the fourchette to the beginning of episiotomy [27, 79], episiotomy angles [24, 27, 43, 45, 46, 47, 79], episiotomy lengths [24, 27, 39, 40, 43, 45, 46, 71, 72, 79]), perineal body lengths in the first [21, 42, 84], second [42] or third [16, 39, 40, 72, 79] stages of labour, range of anal dilation [42]. To reduce the inter-individual variability, a transparent plastic film can be applied to the perineal skin, lines and dots copied onto the film and subsequently measured on a flat plane [24, 27]. However, this step is rather complicated when measurement takes place at the end of the second stage of labour when the exact timing of measurement is of crucial importance. This is also the reason, why experimental studies performing measurements during this short period of time (i.e. when performing an episiotomy, crowning of the fetal head) have been able to evaluate only a limited number of variables.

Application of Direct Measurement on the Perineum in Clinical Practice

Measurement of characteristics of episiotomy (i.e. the beginning of episiotomy, episiotomy angles, episiotomy lengths) facilitated a development of an international classification of episiotomies [44].

Ultrasonography

A second stage of labour ultrasound could be used to diagnose the presence, degree or range of caput succedaneum [32], occipito-posterior presentations [11, 67] or fetal head progression [30, 85]. The distance between the lower margin of the pubic bone and the nearest point on the fetal skull was found to be a reliable method for evaluation of fetal head descent [85] and pubic arch angle measurement may predict the likelihood of instrumental delivery in prolonged second stage of labor [31].

However, there have been no studies performed during the second stage evaluating perineal tension and deformation. The majority of studies focus on levator ani avulsion, the size of levator hiatus or mobility of the ano-rectal junction. There are very few studies evaluating the extent of pre- and postpartum perineal mobility with regards to a variety of obstetric variables. An Australian study found a significantly increased mobility after vaginal delivery, mainly after vacuum-extraction. However, the extent of the mobility did not correlate with the extent of clinically diagnosed perineal trauma [13].

At the moment, ultrasonography is considered to be helpful in the diagnostics of fetal head variables (fetal head size, position, descent). The role of ultrasonography of the perineal body during the final stage of delivery remains to be evaluated. Transperineal/endoanal ultrasound is essential for diagnostic algorithms regarding adverse functional perineal outcome (see Chap. 7).

Magnetic Resonance Imaging (MRI)

At the moment MRI is not well-suited to intrapartum use and so studies tend to focus on evaluating pre- and postpartum anatomy [8, 20, 48, 62]. Moreover, these studies mostly evaluate injury to the levator ani complex [20, 48, 62] rather than the degree of perineal trauma. MR is utilizable in detecting external (EAS) and internal anal sphincter (IAS) injuries postpartum [8] and an improved visualization of EAS atrophy was documented [7]. However, currently, ultrasonography remains the method of choice (see Chap. 7).

Elastography

Elastography is a rapidly developing non-invasive sonographic method that enables assessment of the elasticity and rigidity of various tissues. The method has found its application in a number of medical fields as it allows for the non-invasive examination of mechanical properties of various structures. In obstetrics, elastography of the uterine cervix is studied as a predictor of preterm birth or successful labour induction [57, 59]. Three main methods of tissue elasticity determination have been proposed [29, 63].

1. **Strain elastography.** Compression of the studied tissue, which enables calculation of the relative stiffness of the tissue based on the extent of its movement and deformation. The tissue compression may be performed by the operator or by movement of internal organs (heart, carotid artery, breathing). As this method only enables determination of relative elasticity, it is mainly suitable for the differentiation of solid tumors in soft tissue, e.g. in cases of breast cancer, and is available on most modern advanced ultrasonographs.
2. **Acoustic Radiation Force Impulse Elastography (ARFI)**. The vibration of the examined tissue is induced by acoustic temporal impulse-like excitations and the elasticity of the tissue is determined from transient tissue displacement response within the region of interest. Again, although more sophisticated, it is a qualitative method for elasticity assessment.
3. **Shear-wave elastography**. A quantitative method allowing for the calculation of the elasticity modulus of a tissue area from the speed of propagation of transverse shear waves generated by the probe. The method enables quantitative dynamic evaluation of tissue elasticity within a region of interest. This method is currently under investigation for its potential in the determination of mechanical properties of various tissues; it was demonstrated to be a valid method for the assessment of elasticity modulus of muscular [23, 49], and connective tissue [9]. The method has potential for the assessment of perineal elasticity before or in the course of vaginal delivery. However, at present no device or protocol has been developed for this purpose.

Clinical Perineal Mapping

Clinical perineal mapping is a fast subjective evaluation of the conditions on the perineum during the final moments of the vaginal delivery, i.e. at the time of crowning and expulsion of the fetal head (Fig. 3.4). The variables should be evaluated comprehensively, i.e. as parts of a complex approach to protect the perineal structures since they relate to each other.

The following set of obstetrical variables is commonly evaluated (Table 3.2):

- Size of the fetal head

This variable should correspond with the risk of severe perineal trauma more than expected fetal macrosomia – a recognized risk factor [35, 80]. The size of the fetal head is directly measurable by ultrasonography compared to indirect calculation of the estimated fetal weight. Also, it is the fetal head (and/or fetal shoulders) that bear the highest risk for maternal perineum.

Occipito-posterior position (OPP) is a recognized risk factor of OASIS [26, 66]. In order to reduce the risk of perineal trauma, instrumental delivery or second stage caesarean, some attempts have been made to correct OPP. Maternal positioning during the first stage of labor was studied recently, but the sample size was insufficient to demonstrate clear evidence [81]. There is currently an ongoing trial to re-evaluate this technique [33]. Digital or manual rotation of OPP to occipito-anterior position during the second stage has been suggested with a success rate of 75–93 % [68, 77]. Using this maneuver, the cohort studies reported reduction of instrumental deliveries [68] as well as caesarean sections [77].

Caput succedaneum is an oedema of the subcutaneous layer of the fetal head caused by an obstruction of the venous return, and subsequent extravasation of fluid into the interstitial compartment. Its range is measurable by transperineal ultrasound in case or prolonged second stage of labor [31, 32]. Caput succedaneum started to be evaluated just recently. To our knowledge, effect of caput succedaneum on perineal trauma has never been studied.

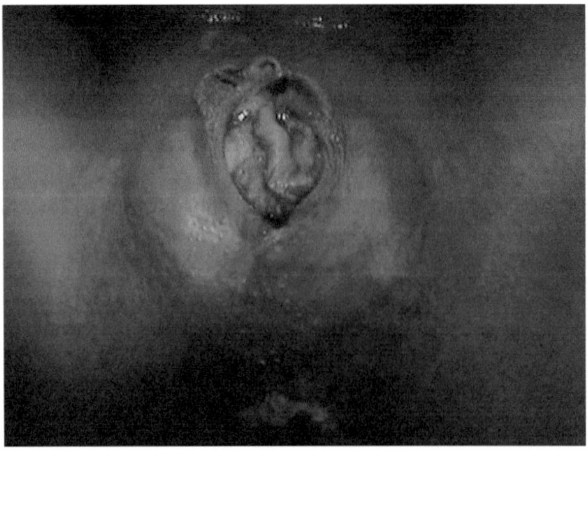

Fig. 3.4 Perineal structures at the end of vaginal delivery

Table 3.2 Obstetric variables analyzed by perineal mapping

Variable	Subvariable	Analyzed by
Size of the fetal head	Fetal macrosomia	External visual assessment
	Occipito-posterior position (OPP)	Transabdominal ultrasonography
	Caput succedaneum	Palpation, identification of bregma, lambda
		Transabdominal, transperineal, transvaginal ultrasonography
Length/diameter of the genital hiatus		External visual assessment
		Direct measurement
Perineal dimensions	Perineal body length	External visual assessment
		Direct measurement
	Anal dilation	External visual assessment
		Direct measurement
Oedema of the perineum		External visual assessment
Tension of the perineal tissues	Elasticity	2nd stage perineal massage, ironing of the perineum
	Incipient perineal tear	Visual observation
		Bleeding
Excessive obstetrical perineal bulging	Degree of fetal flexion/extension	External visual assessment
		Palpation, identification of bregma, lambda
Co-operation of the parturient	Technical approach to the perineum to execute intervention	Verbal rating scale
	Active physical defence of the parturient decreasing the effectiveness of the intervention	Verbal rating scale Presence – absence
	Unexpected pushing	Presence – absence

- Length/diameter of the genital hiatus

According to the International Continence Society, the length (the antero-posterio diameter) of genital hiatus is defined as a distance between the middle of the external urethral meatus and the posterior midline hymen [10]. Because of the shape of the moulded fetal head, during the second stage the dilated vaginal opening is oval [37]. The extent of transverse introital dilation is also important as the transverse strain of perineal structures is four-times higher than antero-posterior deformation [86]. The extent of introital dilation (together with assessment of the fetal head size, elasticity and oedema of the perineum) might facilitate in the decision whether other obstetric interventions are required altogether with their timing (e.g. second stage perineal massage, use of obstetric gel, manual perineal protection, episiotomy).

- Perineal dimensions

Perineal body length (PBL) is commonly measured from the posterior margin of the genital hiatus to the midanal opening [10]. This definition is also used in the majority of studies evaluating the role of this obstetric variable in the development of severe perineal laceration during vaginal delivery [3, 16, 21, 40, 42, 61, 71, 72, 84].

It has been found that the perineal body length does not differ between the different ethnic groups in the first stage of labor and its mean length is 39 mm [21, 84]. A first stage short PBL has occasionally been identified as a risk factor for OASIS [4, 16, 84] while other studies have not found this correlation [21]. A recent international review found reported that a short PBL (<3 cm) was associated with episiotomy [69].

However, in routine the clinical practice, midwives and obstetricians have no information regarding first stage PBL. Nevertheless, the adequate assessment of PBL is possible during the second stage of labour when woman is positioned in lithotomy. It has been shown that the first stage PBL significantly varies from the second stage measurement [42]. Furthermore, because of anal dilation, the second stage PBL ought to be defined as the distance from the fourchette to the border between perianal epidermis and anal squamous epithelium at 12 o'clock from the centre of the anal canal [42] (Fig. 3.2). The mean measured second stage PBL was 50 (range 28–85) mm [42]. Due to the phenomenon of perineal stretching and bulging, the normals for PBL for the first stage of labor are of limited use at the time of crowning. The assessment of the second stage PBL has to be made together with assessment of other perineal characteristics (i.e. anal dilation, oedema, and elasticity). Further studies are needed on evaluation of the second stage PBL and rate and degree of perineal trauma.

Anal dilation is defined as the largest antero-posterior and the largest transverse diameter of visible borders between perianal epidermis and anal epithelium (Fig. 3.2). The mean diameter of anal opening at the end of the second stage of labor is 25 mm [42]. Therefore, anal dilation significantly changes the anthropometric conditions on the perineum during labour. This observation is important mainly in the decision-making process of how an episiotomy should be positioned on the perineum [42].

- Oedema of the perineum

Oedema of the perineum during the final phases of vaginal delivery is a rarely studied variable. In one study, oedema was found a risk factor for OASIS [76]. The risk was higher for higher degree of oedema. Generally, oedematous tissues have a lower elasticity and so higher fragility. Oedema can prolong the passage of the fetus through the pelvic floor structures and could be the result of well-filled pelvis leading to venous congestion caused by a pressure of the fetal head against the pelvic walls resulting in extravasation of fluid into the interstitial space. Theoretically, oedematous perineum can decrease the effectiveness of manual perineal protection applied on the perineal surface.

A thick, inelastic perineum is one of the most common indications for episiotomy [17, 73]. If perineum is substantially oedematous, with non-adequate elasticity, in case with other risk factors (larger fetal head, prolonged second stage of labour), careful execution of episiotomy might become considerable.

- Tension of the perineal tissues

The degree of **elasticity** of the perineum could be, to a certain extent, evaluated by palpation in the second stage of labour. This could be a marker whether perineal tissues are sufficiently elastic and if not whether some interventions (continuing perineal massage, application of warm compresses, slowing the passage of the fetus, waterbirth) might become useful.

Incipient perineal tear is a marker that perineum is excessively stretched and artificial widening of the introitus (episiotomy) averting the vector of the main strain away from the anus is to be fast considered.

- Excessive perineal bulging

The crowning of the fetal head can be defined as an absence in recession of the fetal head between the contractions as parietal eminences have passed the level of ischial spines. At this moment the suboccipit is located at the lower margin of the symphysis pubis while the bregma is situated between the sacrum and coccyx. If the fetal head is not sufficiently and timely extended it continues in its motion away from the pubic symphysis, which excessively bulges the perineal body and results in excessive perineal stretching. In this situation some of the extension methods of manual perineal protection (Ritgen maneuver or Finnish method, see Chap. 4) might become useful to reduce the perineal tension.

- Co-operation of the parturient

The slowing of the passage of the fetus through the perineal structures provides time for relaxation of the tissues. This could be achieved either by a direct pressure of the accoucheur's non-dominant hand on the fetal head [34, 50–53, 56, 58, 79] or by coordinating/guiding the mother to follow instructions to push in a suitable time [34, 50–53, 79]. If the parturient is not capable to co-operate with the attending personnel, she might force the expulsion of the fetal head rapidly and unexpectedly. During such a short period of time the perineum is not given enough time to stretch and the attending personnel cannot perform appropriate manual perineal protection. In a retrospective study inadequate co-operation of the parturient has been shown to be a risk factor for OASIS [40]. However, this variable has to be yet fully evaluated using a better methodological approach.

Perineal Mapping and the Biomechanics of the Manual Perineal Protection During the Expulsion of the Fetal Head

Manual perineal protection (MPP) has been known for about 2000 years [15, 82]. However, due to its variants and complicated reproducibility, this obstetric intervention has not been properly appraised. Throughout the history many expert opinions regarding conduct of the second stage of labour and maneuvers for reduction of peripartum injury have been proposed, occasionally contradicting each other [19] (Table 3.3).

Table 3.3 Classifications of MPP

Classification	Methods	Description
Hands-off, -poised, -on [56, 58]	Hands-off	The expulsion of the fetal head and shoulders is completely unassisted
	Hands-poised	"The accoucheur's hands are poised, and prepared to put light pressure on the baby's head in case of rapid expulsion, otherwise the fetal head or perineum are not touched." Delivery of the shoulders is unassisted as well
	Hands-on	"Accoucheur's hands put pressure on the fetal head in the belief that flexion will be increased, and support ('guard') the perineum. Lateral flexion is used to facilitate the delivery of the shoulders"
Cochrane review [1]	Flexion technique [60] Fig. 3.5	"The accoucheur's hand puts a downward pressure on the fetal occiput towards the perineum to maintain a flexion"
	Original Ritgen maneuver [70] Fig. 3.6	"Three fingers of one hand that hold the head back are placed on the occiput and must not be removed until the head is delivered. Merely tips of four fingers of the other hand are placed on the posterior perineum, behind the anus, in front of the tip of coccyx and slightly laterally. A pressure is directed inside and anteriorly in the period between contractions, at best right after a contraction with the fingers. They will easily meet chin of the child and bring it to a forward motion, while the three fingers on the occiput lead the progression of the head so that the fetal neck leans against the lower margin of the pubis. The two hands should be held still as soon as a contraction starts until it ends. Right after it the pressure on the chin will be resumed. When the head crowns the pressure should continue from the posterior perineum to anus and finally through perineum until the chin passes through the posterior commissure"
	Modified Ritgen maneuver [38]	Ritgen maneuver applied during uterine contractions

Other suggested methods	Central palmar support [19] Fig. 3.7	Using the dominant hand the accoucheur's palm is applied to the perineum in the midline with no co-ordinative work mediated by fingers. Pressure is executed towards the symphysis of pubis. The non-dominant hand controls the rate of the expulsion
	Central digital support [5] Fig. 3.8	The accoucheur's dominant thumb and index-finger exert pressure through the perineum on either side of the anus on the front part of the fetal head and push the head forwards. The non-dominant hand controls the rate of the expulsion
	Viennese technique ([37, 86]; Fig. 3.9	"Accoucheur's dominant thumb and index- or middle-finger are placed alongside the fourchette and vaginal opening. Thumb and index- or middle-finger are squeezed against each other. The area of first dorsal interosseus muscle and the second metacarpo-phalangeal joint may execute a pressure on the fetal forehead to keep the head as close to lower margin of pubis as possible." The non-dominant hand controls the rate of the expulsion
	Finnish technique [50, 51, 65] Fig. 3.10a–c	The dominant thumb and index-finger of the accoucheur are placed alongside the fourchette and vaginal opening. The thumb and index-finger are squeezed against each other. The flexed middle-finger is applied on the posterior perineum and executes an upward pressure to facilitate the extension of the fetal head and keep it as close to the lower margin of the pubis as possible. The non-dominant hand controls the rate of the expulsion and occasionally abets extension of the head

Fig. 3.5 Flexion technique

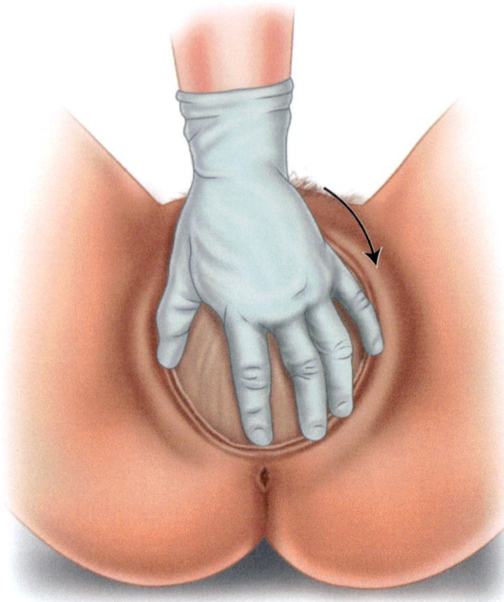

In order to evaluate the manual perineal protection, the classification of the intervention became simplified to hands-off, hands-poised and hands-on techniques [6, 18, 56, 58, 83] (Table 3.3). A recent Cochrane review [1] divided MPP into the flexion technique [60] and Ritgen maneuver [70]. The Ritgen maneuver is further divided into original [70] and modified [38] (Table 3.3).

In the flexion technique, the accoucheur's non-dominant hand applies a pressure to the fetal head on the occipital region behind the lambda (posterior fontanelle) in order to keep the head flexed. It was declared that in this way the fetal head is delivered with its smallest, suboccipito-bregmatic, circumference passing through the birth canal [60] (Fig. 3.5).

The original Ritgen maneuver was published 160 years ago [70]. Briefly described as the tips of four fingers are placed on the perineal skin behind the anus and used to apply forward pressure on the fetal chin to extend the fetal head (Fig. 3.6). However, the Ritgen maneuver is occasionally misinterpreted and thought to be a method where fingers are inserted into the rectum [19], that the pressure is applied to the fetal brow [14] or that the technique is used to maintain head flexion by pressing the fetal chin towards its chest [22]. The full original description translated into English is provided in Table 3.3.

Lacking the technical tools to measure changes in perineal tissue tension during delivery has made it difficult to evaluate the benefit of MPP. In order to overcome these problems the 5P's project (Perineal Protection Program incorporating the Principles of Physics), which is currently ongoing, was introduced to analyse each step of MPP.

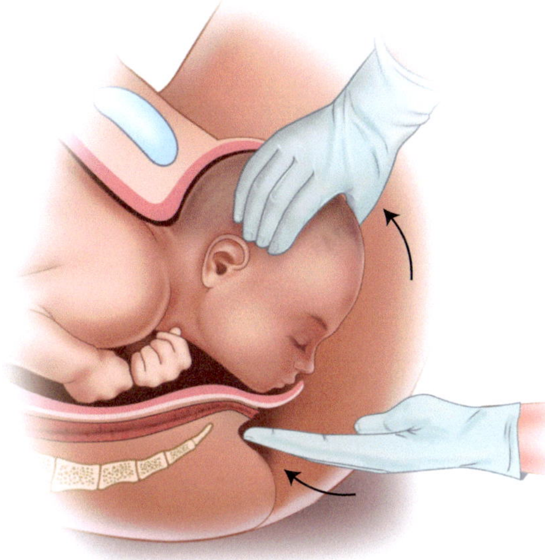

Fig. 3.6 Original Ritgen maneuver

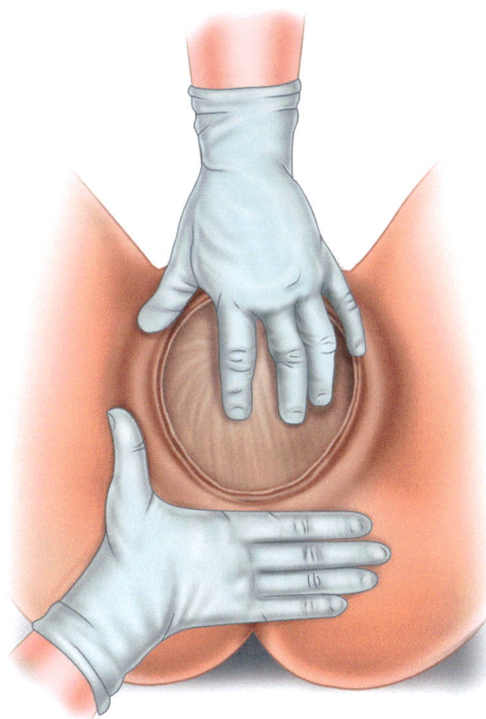

Fig. 3.7 Central palmar support

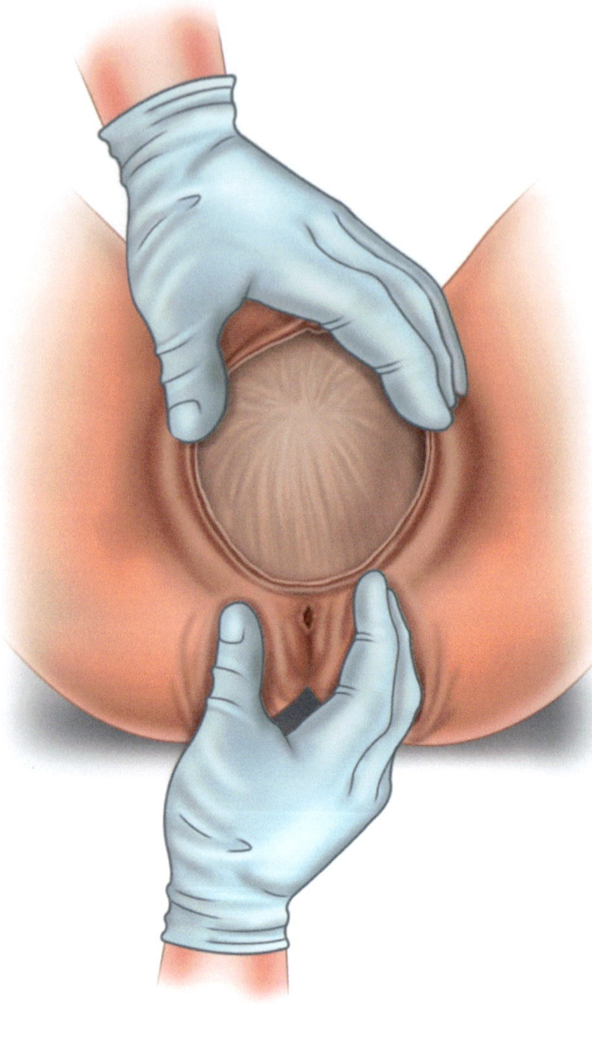

Fig. 3.8 Central digital supports

Based on the principles of mechanics, there are four ways to reduce perineal strain (tension) [86]:

1. Reduction of frictional forces;
2. Increase in the elasticity of the perineum;
3. Dispersal of the perineal tension, i.e. reduction of the perineal tension at its highest point of intensity through its distribution across a larger surface area with regards to transverse tension and antero-posterior tension; and
4. Reduction of effective dimensions of the passing fetal head, i.e. minimization of the maximum head circumference (i.e. the suboccipito-bregmatic circumference) as it passes through the perineal structures.

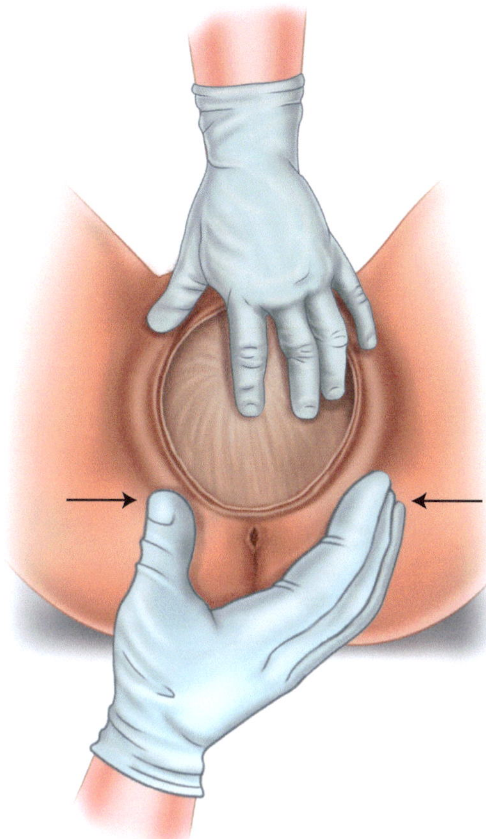

Fig. 3.9 Viennese method

Possible ways to affect frictional forces and elasticity of the perineum are discussed in Chap. 5 (Warm Compresses on the Perineum During Labour and Perineal Massage During Labour).

Dispersal of Perineal Tension

A recent experimental study quantified the changes in strain and deformation of the perineum during the final phase of labour. The highest tissue strain was located at the posterior fourchette. It has been calculated that just before expulsion, the highest tissue strain is in the transverse direction, occurs at the level of the fourchette, and is more than four-times higher than the maximum antero-posterior strain [86]. In the observations, 1 cm of the tissue was transversely stretched and deformed to 2.77 cm during the final stage of vaginal delivery [86].

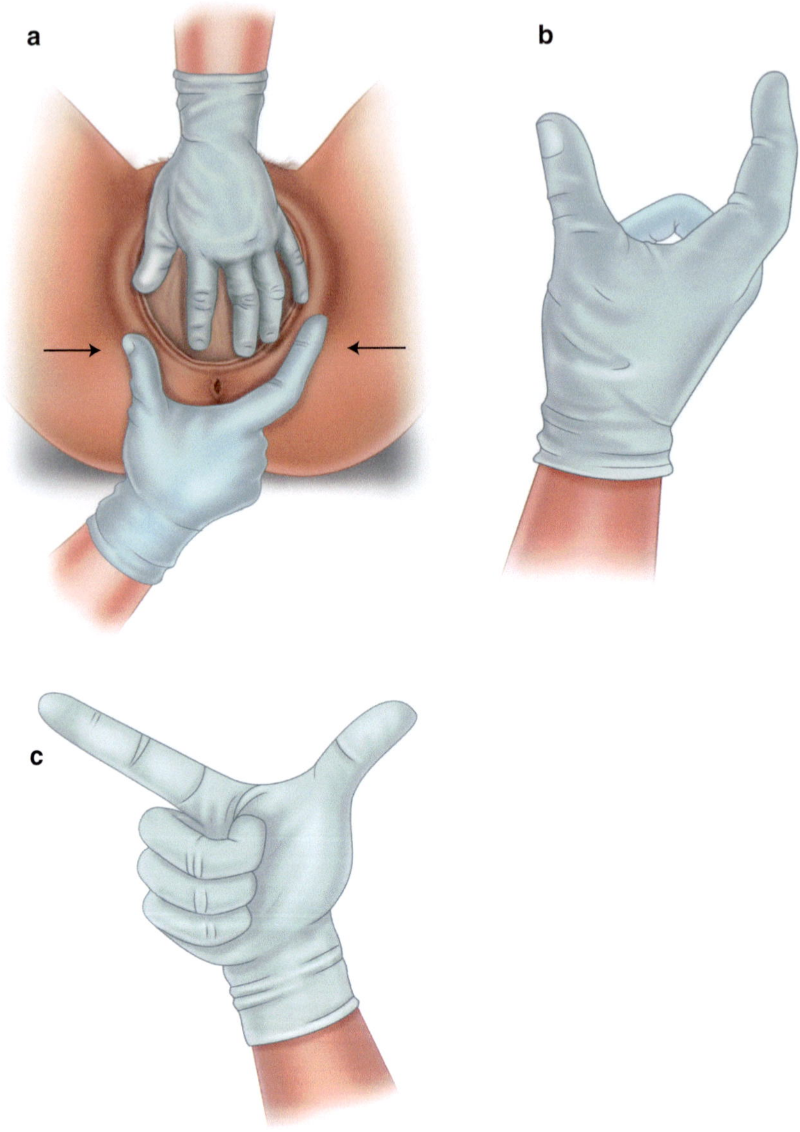

Fig. 3.10 Finnish method. (**a**) Finnish method – application of the accoucheur's hands on the fetal head and perineum; (**b**) Finnish method – accoucheur's dominant hand, view from *above*; (**c**) Finnish method – accoucheur's dominant hand, view from the *front*

Based on this experiment, the traditional Viennese method of protecting the perineum [37, 86] (Table 3.3) was suggested for further testing. A computational quasi-static finite element model was composed (subsection "Virtual Perineal Mapping") based on the initial geometry of the female pelvic floor at the beginning of the second stage of labour and on available data from previous experimental, clinical and biomechanical studies [37]. A biomechanical assessment simulating vaginal delivery both with and without MPP showed that, based on biomechanical principles, the appropriate application of the thumb and the index-finger of the accoucheur's dominant hand on the perineal skin during the second stage of labour considerably reduces the tissue tension throughout the entire perineal body thickness. Therefore, this intervention might be beneficial in reducing the rate and/or degree of the obstetric perineal injury [37].

Further testing found that the exact positioning of the fingers and their subsequent co-ordinated work plays an important role in the extent of the reduction of the maximum tension [37]. To perform MPP effectively, the fingers must be placed sufficiently anteriorly and apart, and follow the vector of the principal perineal strain. If the positioning of the fingers moves away from this vector, the effectiveness of MPP is substantially reduced. In the best modification of the Viennese method of MPP in the delivery of an average-sized fetal head, the initial position of the fingers was 12 cm apart and 2 cm anteriorly from the posterior fourchette with a bilateral movement of 1 cm towards the midline with no movement in the antero-posterior dimension (see Fig. 3.11) [37]. This test also showed that a distance of 1 cm in the wrong direction is responsible for nearly a 30 % difference in the maximum perineal tension [37] (Fig. 3.11).

Further experimentation revealed that the Viennese method markedly reduces the perineal tension for various sizes of the fetal head and that the modification(s) most effective in reducing the perineal tension for an average-sized head remained

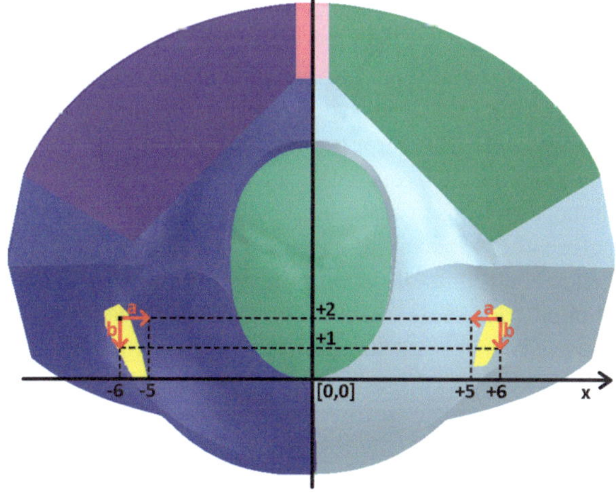

Fig. 3.11 Application and subsequent movement of fingers in the best modification of Viennese method (a), compared to movement of fingers in a wrong direction (b)

the most efficient for the delivery of substantially smaller or larger infants [41]. It has also been shown that the exact execution of the best modification of MPP during the delivery of macrosomic infants might reduce the perineal tension to below the strain achieved when using the "hands-off" technique for a small fetus [41]. This supports the concept that the most effective MPP should be easily acquirable, clinically practical and routinely provided. The authors believe that MPP should be executed for the delivery of all infants, not only reserved for fetal macrosomia.

Decreasing the Size of the Passing Object

Both flexion and extension techniques have been devised to achieve passing of the shortest circumference of the fetal head through the structures of the perineum [60]. However, it is obvious that these techniques are mechanically opposing.

During a normal birth, no intervention is required until the crowning of the fetal head. As the flexed head progresses downwards, the smallest, suboccipito-bregmatic circumference is passing through the pelvis.

During the natural course of labour, from crowning, the head must be transformed from flexion into extension. This may happen either spontaneously or with assistance.

Considering the physiological anatomy of the female pelvis and the natural course of the vaginal delivery it is evident that if the flexion technique is continuously and persistently performed, this technique will only cause excessive ill-calculated posterior pressure against the perineum and expose the perineum to inadequate redundant strain.

Spontaneous sufficient extension of the crowning fetal head depends on the anatomical dimensions and material properties of the perineum and whether the perineum provides the sufficient resistance needed to direct the head anteriorly to pivot around the lower margin of the pubic bone. However, the dimensions and material properties of the perineal tissues are highly variable between individuals and are not known with any precision. More importantly, they are not measurable at the time of vaginal delivery in everyday clinical practice. Therefore, the extent of natural spontaneous extension remains uncertain. Furthermore, considering the effectiveness of the appropriate modification of the Viennese method, the natural course of the delivery might be altered by this technique. In this Viennese technique, as well as in any modification of MPP, the fingers are placed on the perineum before the suboccipito-bregmatic circumference passes through the perineum, hence before the extension of fetal head is completed. Since the fingers have to be applied effectively to the skin, a considerable pressure through the perineal skin caused by applying the fingertips deeper towards the parietal bones of the fetal head is developed (see Fig. 3.12). This pressure may, at least in some cases, alter the natural course of the final extension the fetal head and keep the head flexed even at the time of its expulsion. Based on this biomechanical reasoning, some modification of manual/digital assistance to extend the crowning fetal head ought to decrease the dimension of the passing circumference of the fetal head. All

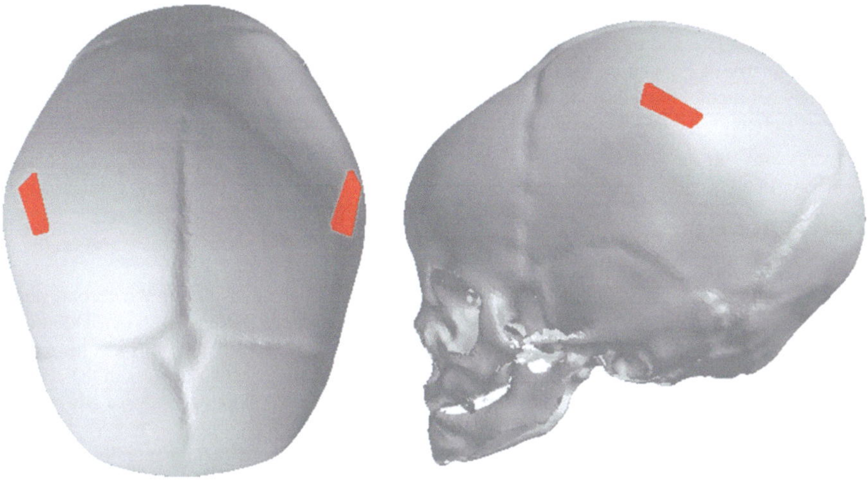

Fig. 3.12 Imprints of the fingers on the fetal head at the initiation of MPP (best modification) with regards to position of bregma (anterior fontanelle)

Norwegian studies used the Finnish technique to support the perineum [34, 50, 51, 53, 78, 79]. In this technique a flexed middle finger facilitates the final extension of the fetal head (see Fig. 3.10).

Conclusion

Perineal mapping has been found to be a modern effective tool in the analysis of obstetric interventions that have previously lacked a sufficient quality of evidence as their precise execution could not be controlled. By means of experimental perineal mapping a variety of hurdles in obtaining ethical approval can be bypassed and the methodological inaccuracies of recent clinical studies can be revealed. Furthermore, based on biomechanical principles, perineal mapping can explain why these clinical studies failed, can be used to analyse impact of complex obstetric interventions separately and suggest the appropriate multifaceted clinical approach.

To facilitate advances in research in this field, mere standardisation of the methodology of reporting trials is not sufficient. The precise description of the technique itself is of paramount importance in order to establish a common platform for research. Further improvements expected in the field of computational modeling may assist in performing appropriate assessments of other obstetric interventions. Indeed, future progress may result in the development of complex computational or physical tools [54] where a variety of obstetric interventions and their modifications might be tested and quantitatively compared in order to achieve a uniform language and true understanding of such a complex process as vaginal birth.

Acknowledgments The work on this chapter was supported by the Charles University Research Fund (Progres Q39) and by the National Sustainability Program I (NPU I) Nr. LO1503 provided by the Ministry of Education, Youth and Sports of the Czech Republic and by the project SGS-2016-059 (Computer modeling and monitoring of human body used for medicine) of the University of West Bohemia.

References

1. Aasheim V, Nilsen AB, Lukasse M, Reinar LM. Perineal techniques during the second stage of labour for reducing perineal trauma. Cochrane Database Syst Rev. 2011;12:CD006672. doi:10.1002/14651858.CD006672.pub2.
2. Albers LL, Sedler KD, Bedrick EJ, Teaf D, Peralta P. Midwifery care measures in the second stage of labor and reduction of genital tract trauma at birth: a randomized trial. J Midwifery Womens Health. 2005;50:365–72.
3. Andrews V, Thakar R, Sultan AH, Jones PW. Are mediolateral episiotomies actually mediolateral? BJOG. 2005;112:1156–8.
4. Aytan H, Tapisiz OL, Tuncay G, Avsar FA. Severe perineal lacerations in nulliparous women and episiotomy type. Eur J Obstet Gynecol Reprod Biol. 2005;121(1):46–50.
5. Baker PN, Monga A. Obstetric procedures. Normal labour. In: Obstetrics by ten teachers. London: Arnold; 1995. p. 183.
6. Berghella V, Baxter JK, Chauhan SP. Evidence-based labor and delivery management. Am J Obstet Gynecol. 2008;199:445–54.
7. Bharucha AE, Fletcher JG, Harper CM, Hough D, Daube JR, Stevens C, Seide B, Riederer SJ, Zinsmeister AR. Relationship between symptoms and disordered continence mechanisms in women with idiopathic faecal incontinence. Gut. 2005;54(4):546–55.
8. Bharucha AE, Fletcher JG, Melton 3rd LJ, Zinsmeister AR. Obstetric trauma, pelvic floor injury and fecal incontinence: a population-based case-control study. Am J Gastroenterol. 2012;107(6):902–11.
9. Brum J, Bernal M, Gennisson JL, Tanter M. In vivo evaluation of the elastic anisotropy of the human Achilles tendon using shear wave dispersion analysis. Phys Med Biol. 2014;59(3):505–23. doi:10.1088/0031-9155/59/3/505.
10. Bump RC, Mattiasson A, Bo K, Brubaker LP, DeLancey JOL, Klarskov P, et al. The standardization of terminology of female pelvic organ prolapse and pelvic floor dysfunction. Am J Obstet Gynecol. 1996;175:10–7.
11. Carseldine WJ, Phipps H, Zawada SF, Campbell NT, Ludlow JP, Krishnan SY, De Vries BS. Does occiput posterior position in the second stage of labour increase the operative delivery rate? Aust N Z J Obstet Gynaecol. 2013;53(3):265–70.
12. Chaliha C, Sultan AH, Bland JM, Monga AK, Stanton SL. Anal function: effect of pregnancy and delivery. Am J Obstet Gynecol. 2001;185(2):427–32.
13. Chantarasorn V, Shek KL, Dietz HP. Mobility of the perineal body and anorectal junction before and after childbirth. Int Urogynecol J. 2012;23(6):729–33.
14. Cunningham FG. The Ritgen maneuver: another sacred cow questioned. Obstet Gynecol. 2008;112(2 Pt 1):210–1.
15. Dahlen HG, Homer CS, Leap N, Tracy SK. From social to surgical: historical perspectives on perineal care during labour and birth. Women Birth. 2011;24(3):105–11.
16. Deering SH, Carlson N, Stitely M, Allaire AD, Satin AJ. Perineal body length and lacerations at delivery. J Reprod Med. 2004;49(4):306–10.
17. de Oliveira SM, Miquilini EC. Frequency and criteria for the indication of episiotomy. Rev Esc Enferm USP. 2005;39(3):288–95.
18. de Souza Caroci da Costa A, Gonzalez Riesco ML. A comparison of "hands off" versus "hands on" techniques for decreasing perineal lacerations during birth. J Midwifery Womens Health. 2006;51(2):106–11.

19. DeWees WB. Relaxation and management of the perineum during parturition. J Am Med Assoc. 1889;24:841–8.
20. Dietz HP, Gillespie AV, Phadke P. Avulsion of the pubovisceral muscle associated with large vaginal tear after normal vaginal delivery at term. Aust N Z J Obstet Gynaecol. 2007;47(4):341–4.
21. Dua A, Whitworth M, Dugdale A, Hill S. Perineal length: norms in gravid women in the first stage of labour. Int Urogynecol J Pelvic Floor Dysfunct. 2009;20(11):1361–4. doi:10.1007/s00192-009-0959-x.
22. Eason E, Labrecque M, Wells G, Feldman P. Preventing perineal trauma during childbirth: a systematic review. Obstet Gynecol. 2000;95(3):464–71.
23. Eby SF, Song P, Chen S, Chen Q, Greenleaf JF, An KN. Validation of shear wave elastography in skeletal muscle. J Biomech. 2013;46(14):2381–7. doi:10.1016/j.jbiomech.2013.07.033.
24. Eogan M, Daly L, O'Connell P, O'Herlihy C. Does the angle of episiotomy affect the incidence of anal sphincter injury? BJOG. 2006;113:190–4.
25. Falk-Larsen J, Schmidt T. Klinisk Obstetrik. København: Munksgaard; 1983. p. 79–80.
26. Fitzpatrick M, McQuillan K, O'Herlihy C. Influence of persistent occiput posterior position on delivery outcome. Obstet Gynecol. 2001;98(6):1027–31.
27. Fodstad K, Laine K, Staff AC. Different episiotomy techniques, postpartum perineal pain, and blood loss: an observational study. Int Urogynecol J. 2013;24(5):865–72.
28. Fung YC. Biomechanics – mechanical properties of living tissues. 2nd ed. New York: Springer; 1993.
29. Garra BS. Imaging and estimation of tissue elasticity by ultrasound. Ultrasound Q. 2007;23(4):255–68.
30. Ghi T, Youssef A, Maroni E, Arcangeli T, De Musso F, Bellussi F, Nanni M, Giorgetta F, Morselli-Labate AM, Iammarino MT, Paccapelo A, Cariello L, Rizzo N, Pilu G. Intrapartum transperineal ultrasound assessment of fetal head progression in active second stage of labor and mode of delivery. Ultrasound Obstet Gynecol. 2013;41(4):430–5.
31. Gilboa Y, Kivilevitch Z, Spira M, Kedem A, Katorza E, Moran O, Achiron R. Pubic arch angle in prolonged second stage of labor: clinical significance. Ultrasound Obstet Gynecol. 2013;41(4):442–6.
32. Gilboa Y, Kivilevitch Z, Kedem A, Spira M, Borkowski T, Moran O, Katorza E, Achiron R. Caput succedaneum thickness in prolonged second stage of labour: a clinical evaluation. Aust N Z J Obstet Gynaecol. 2013;53(5):459–63. doi:10.1111/ajo.12104.
33. Guittier MJ, Othenin-Girard V, Irion O, Boulvain M. Maternal positioning to correct occipito-posterior fetal position in labour: a randomised controlled trial. BMC Pregnancy Childbirth. 2014;14(1):83. doi:10.1186/1471-2393-14-83.
34. Hals E, Øian P, Pirhonen T, Gissler M, Hjelle S, Nilsen EB, et al. A multicenter interventional program to reduce the incidence of anal sphincter tears. Obstet Gynecol. 2010;116(4):901–8. doi:10.1097/AOG.0b013e3181eda77a.
35. Handa VL, Danielsen BH, Gilbert WM. Obstetric anal sphincter lacerations. Obstet Gynecol. 2001;98(2):225–30.
36. Jansova M, Kalis V, Lobovsky L, Hyncik L, Karbanova J, Rusavy Z. The role of thumb and index-finger placement in manual perineal protection. Int Urogynecol J. 2014;25(11):1533–40. doi:10.1007/s00192-014-2425-7.
37. Jansova M, Kalis V, Rusavy Z, Zemcik R, Lobovsky L, Laine K. Modeling manual perineal protection during vaginal delivery. Int Urogynecol J. 2014;25(1):65–71. přidat doi10.10 07s00192-013-2164-1.
38. Jönsson ER, Elfaghi I, Rydhström H, Herbst A. Modified Ritgen's maneuver for anal sphincter injury at delivery: a randomized controlled trial. Obstet Gynecol. 2008;112(2 Pt 1):212–7.
39. Kalis V, Chaloupka P, Turek J, Rokyta Z. Risk factors for 3rd and 4th degree perineal ruptures during delivery. Ceska Gynekol. 2005;70(1):30–6.
40. Kalis V, Chaloupka P, Turek J, Rokyta Z. The perineal body length and injury at delivery. Ceska Gynekol. 2005;70(5):355–61.
41. Kalis V, Jansova M, Lobovsky L, Hyncik L, Karbanova J, Rusavy Z. Correct execution of manual perineal protection and the size of the fetal head. 14 AUGS/IUGA Scientific Meeting. 2014. Podium presentation No. 16.

42. Kalis V, Karbanova J, Bukacova Z, Bednarova B, Rokyta Z, Kralickova M. Anal dilation during labor. Int J Gynaecol Obstet. 2010;109(2):136–9. doi:10.1016/j.ijgo.2009.11.024.
43. Kalis V, Karbanova J, Horak M, Lobovsky L, Kralickova M, Rokyta Z. The incision angle of mediolateral episiotomy before delivery and after repair. Int J Gynaecol Obstet. 2008;103(1):5–8.
44. Kalis V, Laine K, de Leeuw JW, Ismail KM, Tincello DG. Classification of episiotomy: towards a standardisation of terminology. BJOG. 2012;119(5):522–6.
45. Kalis V, Ladsmanova J, Bednarova B, Karbanova J, Laine K, Rokyta Z. Evaluation of the incision angle of mediolateral episiotomy at 60 degrees. Int J Gynaecol Obstet. 2011;112(3):220–4. doi:10.1016/j.ijgo.2010.09.015.
46. Kalis V, Stepan Jr J, Horak M, Roztocil A, Kralickova M, Rokyta Z. Definitions of mediolateral episiotomy in Europe. Int J Gynaecol Obstet. 2008;100(2):188–9.
47. Karbanova J, Landsmanova J, Novotny Z. The angle of mediolateral episiotomy using ischial tuberosity as a reference point. Int J Gynaecol Obstet. 2009;107(2):157.
48. Kearney R, Miller JM, Ashton-Miller JA, DeLancey JO. Obstetric factors associated with levator ani muscle injury after vaginal birth. Obstet Gynecol. 2006;107(1):144–9.
49. Koo TK, Guo JY, Cohen JH, Parker KJ. Quantifying the passive stretching response of human tibialis anterior muscle using shear wave elastography. Clin Biomech (Bristol, Avon). 2014;29(1):33–9. doi:10.1016/j.clinbiomech.2013.11.009.
50. Laine K, Gissler M, Pirhonen J. Changing incidence of anal sphincter tears in four Nordic countries through the last decades. Eur J Obstet Gynecol Reprod Biol. 2009;146(1):71–5.
51. Laine K, Pirhonen T, Rolland R, Pirhonen J. Decreasing the incidence of anal sphincter tears during delivery. Obstet Gynecol. 2008;111(5):1053–7. doi:10.1097/AOG.0b013e31816c4402.
52. Laine K, Rotvold W, Staff AC. Are obstetric anal sphincter ruptures preventable? – large and consistent rupture rate variations between the Nordic countries and between delivery units in Norway. Acta Obstet Gynecol Scand. 2013;92(1):94–100.
53. Laine K, Skjeldestad FE, Sandvik L, Staff AC. Incidence of obstetric anal sphincter injuries after training to protect the perineum: cohort study. BMJ Open. 2012;2(5). pii: e001649. doi: 10.1136/bmjopen-2012-001649.
54. Lavesson T, Griph ID, Skarvad A, Karlsson A, Nilsson HB, Steinvall M, Haadem K. A perineal protection device designed to protect the perineum during 3 labor: a multicenter randomized controlled. Eur J Obstet Gynecol. 2014. http://dx.doi.org/10.1016/j.ejogrb.2014.07.006.
55. Li X, Kruger JA, Nash MP, Nielsen PM. Modeling childbirth: elucidating the mechanisms of labor. Wiley Interdiscip Rev Syst Biol Med. 2010;2(4):460–70.
56. Mayerhofer K, Bodner-Adler B, Bodner K, Rabl M, Kaider A, Wagenbichler P, et al. Traditional care of the perineum during birth. A prospective, randomized, multicenter study of 1,076 women. J Reprod Med. 2002;47:477–82.
57. Mazza E, Parra-Saavedra M, Bajka M, Gratacos E, Nicolaides K, Deprest J. In vivo assessment of the biomechanical properties of the uterine cervix in pregnancy. Prenat Diagn. 2014;34(1):33–41.
58. McCandlish R, Bowler U, van Asten H, Berridge G, Winter C, Sames L, et al. A randomised controlled trial of care of the perineum during second stage of normal labour. Br J Obstet Gynaecol. 1998;105(12):1262–72.
59. Molina FS, Gómez LF, Florido J, Padilla MC, Nicolaides KH. Quantification of cervical elastography: a reproducibility study. Ultrasound Obstet Gynecol. 2012;39(6):685–9. doi:10.1002/uog.11067.
60. Myrfield K, Brook C, Creedy D. Reducing perineal trauma: implications of flexion and extension of the fetal head during birth. Midwifery. 1997;13(4):197–201.
61. Nager CW, Helliwell JP. Episiotomy increases perineal laceration length in primiparous women. Am J Obstet Gynecol. 2001;185(2):444–50.
62. Otcenasek M, Krofta L, Baca V, Grill R, Kucera E, Herman H, Vasicka I, Drahonovsky J, Feyereisl J. Bilateral avulsion of the puborectal muscle: magnetic resonance imaging-based three-dimensional reconstruction and comparison with a model of a healthy nulliparous woman. Ultrasound Obstet Gynecol. 2007;29(6):692–6.

63. Palmeri ML, Nightingale KR. Acoustic radiation force-based elasticity imaging methods. Interface Focus. 2011:rsfs20110023.
64. Parnell C, Langhoff-Roos J, Møller H. Conduct of labor and rupture of the sphincter ani. Acta Obstet Gynecol Scand. 2001;80:256–61.
65. Pirhonen JP, Grenman SE, Haadem K, Gudmundsson S, Lindqvist P, Siihola S, et al. Frequency of anal sphincter rupture at delivery in Sweden and Finland – result of difference in manual help to the baby's head. Acta Obstet Gynecol Scand. 1998;77(10):974–7.
66. Ponkey SE, Cohen AP, Heffner LJ, Liberman E. Persistent fetal occiput posterior position: obstetrics outcome. Obstet Gynecol. 2003;101(5 Pt 1):915–20.
67. Ramphul M, Kennelly M, Murphy DJ. Establishing the accuracy and acceptability of abdominal ultrasound to define the foetal head position in the second stage of labour: a validation study. Eur J Obstet Gynecol Reprod Biol. 2012;164(1):35–9.
68. Reichman O, Gdansky E, Latinsky B, Labi S, Samueloff A. Digital rotation from occipito-posterior to occipito-anterior decreases the need for cesarean section. Eur J Obstet Gynecol Reprod Biol. 2008;136(1):25–8.
69. Riethmuller D, Courtois L, Maillet R. Liberal versus restrictive practice of episiotomy: do there exist specific obstetrical indications for episiotomy? J Gynecol Obstet Biol Reprod (Paris). 2006;35(1 Suppl):1S32–9.
70. Ritgen G. Ueber sein Dammschutzverfahren. Monatschrift fur Geburtskunde u Frauenkrankh. 1855;6:321–47.
71. Rizk DE, Abadir MN, Thomas LB, Abu-Zidan F. Determinants of the length of episiotomy or spontaneous posterior perineal lacerations during vaginal birth. Int Urogynecol J Pelvic Floor Dysfunct. 2005;16(5):395–400.
72. Rizk DE, Thomas L. Relationship between the length of the perineum and position of the anus and vaginal delivery in primigravidae. Int Urogynecol J Pelvic Floor Dysfunct. 2000;11(2):79–83.
73. Rusavy Z, Kalis V, Landsmanova J, Kasova L, Karbanova J, Dolejsova K, Sykora T, Necesalova P, Novotny Z. Perineal audit: reasons for more than one thousand episiotomies. Ceska Gynekol. 2011;76(5):378–85.
74. Sackett DL. Evidence-based medicine and treatment choices. Lancet. 1997;349(9051):570.
75. Sackett DL, Richardson WS, Rosenberg W, Haynes RB. Evidence-based medicine. How to practice and teach EBM. New York: Churchill Livingstone; 1997.
76. Samuelsson E, Ladfors L, Wennerholm UB, Gareberg B, Nyberg K, Hagberg H. Anal sphincter tears: prospective study of obstetric risk factors. BJOG. 2000;107:926–31.
77. Schaffer BL, Cheng YW, Vargas JE, Laros Jr RK, Caughey AB. Manual rotation of the fetal occiput: predictors of success and delivery. Am J Obstet Gynecol. 2006;194(5):e7–9.
78. Stedenfeldt M, Øian P, Gissler M, Blix E, Pirhonen J. Risk factors for obstetric anal sphincter injury after a successful multicentre interventional programme. BJOG. 2014;121(1):83–91. doi:10.1111/1471-0528.12274.
79. Stedenfeldt M, Pirhonen J, Blix E, Wilsgaard T, Vonen B, Øian P. Episiotomy characteristics and risks for obstetric anal sphincter injuries: a case-control study. BJOG. 2012;119(6):724–30.
80. Stotland NE, Caughey AB, Breed EM, Escobar GJ. Risk factors and obstetric complications associated with macrosomia. Int J Gynaecol Obstet. 2004;87(3):220–6.
81. Stremler R, Hodnett E, Petryshen P, Stevens B, Weston J, Willan AR. Randomized controlled trial of hands-and-knees positioning for occipitoposterior position in labor. Birth. 2005;32(4):243–51.
82. Temkin O. Soranus' gynaecology. Baltimore: The Johns Hopkins University Press; 1956.
83. Trochez R, Waterfield M, Freeman RM. Hands on or hands off the perineum: a survey of care of the perineum in labour (HOOPS). Int Urogynecol J. 2011;22:1279–85.
84. Tsai PJ, Oyama IA, Hiraoka M, Minaglia S, Thomas J, Kaneshiro B. Perineal body length among different racial groups in the first stage of labor. Female Pelvic Med Reconstr Surg. 2012;18(3):165–7. doi:10.1097/SPV.0b013e318255b096.

85. Youssef A, Maroni E, Ragusa A, De Musso F, Salsi G, Iammarino MT, Paccapelo A, Rizzo N, Pilu G, Ghi T. Fetal head-symphysis distance: a simple and reliable ultrasound index of fetal head station in labor. Ultrasound Obstet Gynecol. 2013;41(4):419–24.
86. Zemčík R, Karbanova J, Kalis V, Lobovsky L, Jansova J, Rusavy Z. Stereophotogrammetry of the perineum during vaginal delivery. Int J Gynaecol Obstet. 2012;109(2):136–9.
87. Zienkiewicz OC, Taylor RL, Zhu JZ. The finite element method: its basis and fundamentals. 6th ed. Butterworth-Heinemann; 2005. ISBN 0750663200.

Chapter 4
Risk Factors for Perineal Trauma

Jan Willem de Leeuw, Sari Räisänen, and Katariina Laine

Abstract Trauma to the perineum may inevitably occur during vaginal delivery. Smaller perineal trauma, without involvement of the anal sphincter muscles, usually has no long term sequelae. Ruptures of the anal sphincters, however, may predispose to the development of anal incontinence in later life and should therefore be avoided.

Knowledge of risk factors that may increase the risk of anal sphincter injuries (OASIS) may help to reduce the number of these injuries, but unfortunately most of these factors are, non-modifiable. Examples of these factors are nulliparity, duration of second stage of labour, high fetal birth weight, abnormal fetal presentation, previous OASIS or caesarean section.

The only direct modifiable risk factor for OASIS during delivery is the choice of instrument in case of operative vaginal delivery. In this, the use of vacuum extraction carries a significantly lower risk than the use of a forceps.

The importance of each risk factor is not solely dependent on the associated risk of trauma but depends also on the prevalence of each factor. For instance, nulliparity is probably the most common risk factor for OASIS, hence, a major risk factor for complex perineal trauma. However, it is important to realise that the vast majority of OASIS occur in women with a priori a relatively low risk. This implies that

J.W. de Leeuw (✉)
Ikazia Hospital, Rotterdam, The Netherlands
e-mail: jw.de.leeuw@ikazia.nl

S. Räisänen
University of Helsinki, Helsinki, Finland
e-mail: shraisanen@gmail.com

K. Laine
Oslo University Hospital, Ullevål, Norway
Department of Obstetrics, University of Oslo, Oslo, Norway
e-mail: kattiksen@yahoo.no

K.M.K. Ismail (ed.), *Perineal Trauma at Childbirth*,
DOI 10.1007/978-3-319-14860-1_4

it is important that during every delivery the supervising obstetrician or midwife offers risk reducing interventions to the delivering woman, as will be explained in Chap. 5.

Keywords Parity • Vacuum extraction • Forceps delivery • Anal sphincter injury

Introduction

It is inevitable that during vaginal delivery trauma to the perineum may occur.

Most commonly the extent of perineal trauma is classified according to the RCOG classification suggested by Sultan [1] (Table 4.1).

In contrast to third and fourth degree ruptures [collectively known as Obstetric Anal Sphincter Injuries (OASIS)], first and second degree perineal tears are not considered to be a cause of long term sequelae as faecal incontinence.

OASIS is the most important risk factor for female anal incontinence. Prevention of high-grade complex perineal trauma is therefore of paramount importance.

Undoubtedly, recognition of risk factors for OASIS is the first step in its prevention. Based on this recognition, it is of paramount importance that birth attendants should be aware of the presence of such risk factors in an individual women and take these into consideration when making decisions in an attempt to prevent or at least mitigate their background risk for OASIS. Unfortunately, many important risk factors are non-modifiable or avoidable, e.g. first vaginal birth. Moreover, the majority of complex perineal trauma happens to women considered to be "low risk". Therefore, it is essential that every supervising obstetrician or midwife is able to undertake measures to prevent OASIS even in women considered to be at low risk for this type of trauma.

It is important to recognise that establishment of the currently known risk factors for OASIS is based on large population studies that have the power to discriminate between the associations of different risk factors with regard to the relatively uncommon outcome of OASIS.

Table 4.1 Classification of perineal ruptures according to [1]

Degree of perineal rupture	
First degree	Injury to perineal skin and/or vaginal mucosa
Second degree	Injury to perineum involving perineal muscles but not involving sthe anal sphincter
Third-degree	Injury to perineum involving the anal sphincter complex
Grade 3a	Less than 50 % of external anal sphincter thickness torn
Grade 3b	More than 50 % of external anal sphincter thickness torn
Grade 3c	Both external and internal anal sphincter torn
Fourth-degree	Injury to perineum involving the complete thickness of the anal sphincter complex and anorectal mucosa

In this chapter we present the most important risk factors for the occurrence of serious perineal trauma.

Parity

In virtually all studies concerning risk factors for serious perineal trauma, nulliparity is identified as one of the major risk factor for OASIS.

All these studies used multivariate analysis for the calculation of the individual risk factors with correction for many other obstetrical variables as fetal birth weight, mode of delivery, fetal position or duration of second stage of labour.

A large population based study using data from Californian hospitals with more than two million deliveries in the database showed that multiparous women had a much lower risk for OASIS compared to nulliparous women [2]. Several European population based studies corroborated the results of this study. In a study from the Netherlands using a national obstetric database containing almost 285,000 deliveries, a more than doubled risk for nulliparous women to sustain OASIS was found, a finding similarly confirmed by a large population based study from Finland [3, 4]. In a Norwegian study describing more than 1.6 million deliveries from 1967 to 2004, a much higher risk for nulliparous women delivering vaginally compared to multiparous women was described and this risk declined with each following delivery up to the sixth vaginal delivery [5]. The increased risk for nulliparous women is usually explained by the relative inelasticity of the perineum. It is also possible that with increasing parity, the vaginal outlet may be even wider resulting in decreasing risk for such complex trauma.

It is important to highlight that in the context of parity and perineal trauma it is more accurate to consider 1st vaginal birth rather than nulliparity. This is particularly relevant with the drive towards increasing vaginal birth after caesarean section (VBAC). Women having their 1st VBAC are by definition not nulliparous, nevertheless, they share the same risk profile for perineal trauma as a nulliparous woman aiming for a vaginal birth. Indeed their risk may be even higher due to the potential confounding effect of increasing fetal birth weight with parity (see section "Previous Delivery by Cesarean Section").

Fetal Birth Weight

Fetal birth weight is associated with the risk for OASIS in almost every study on this subject. Several studies have studied fetal birth weight as a dichotomous variable with a fixed cut-off level.

An American study showed that a fetal birth weight of more than 4000 g was associated with a more than doubled risk for sphincter lesions during delivery (OR 2.17, 95 % CI: 2.07–2.27) [2].

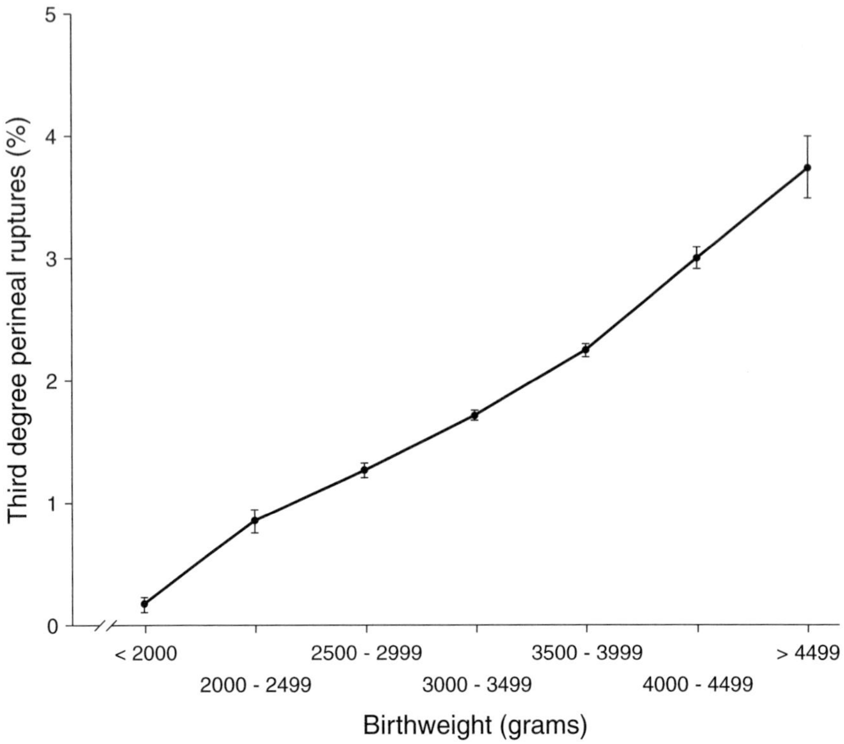

Fig. 4.1 Risk of third degree perineal ruptures per 500 g birth weight (Reprinted from de Leeuw et al. [3] with permission from John Wiley and Sons, Inc.)

In the Norwegian population based study, fetal birth weight was studied with a subdivision of the cohort in groups of 500 g increment of the fetal birth weight with the group of women delivering babies with birth weights between 3000 and 3499 g serving as the reference group. Birth weights of 2500–2999 g and <2500 g were associated with 50 % and 80 % lower risk for sustaining an OASIS respectively [5]. In contrast, increasing birth weight was associated with a significantly higher risk for OASIS with a more than fourfold increased risk for women delivering a baby with a weight of 4500–4999 g. These results were corroborated by several other European studies. Fetal birthweight showed an almost linear association with the risk of OASIS in a Dutch population based study (Fig. 4.1) [3].

Studies addressing parity as a possible risk factor for nulli- and multiparous women separately found similar results [4, 6]. In all subgroups fetal birthweight appeared to be a stronger risk factor in multiparous women than in nulliparous women. Possibly, the risk associated with parity itself outweighs the risk of fetal birthweight leading to a weaker association of fetal birthweight in nulliparous women.

Almost all other studies on this subject have shown, with varying odds, that fetal birth weight is associated with an increased risk for OASIS. In this, one must bear in mind that all studies have used the actual fetal birthweight, established after delivery.

In daily practice, it will be the challenge to rely on estimated fetal birthweight to make a reliable calculation of the expected risk of OASIS during vaginal delivery.

Mode of Delivery

With regard to the risk of damage of the perineum during birth, the method of delivery is one of the most important issues to address.

To address the risk of the various methods a comparison has to be made between spontaneous vaginal delivery versus operative vaginal delivery, and between the different types of operative vaginal delivery, i.e. vacuum and forceps delivery.

In European population based studies operative vaginal deliveries were associated with an increased risk for OASIS compared to spontaneous vaginal deliveries. The risk for OASIS doubled with the use of vacuum extraction and was fourfold when the baby was delivered with the help of forceps [3, 4].

Studies from other continents showed similar results. Ampt et al. described a population based study from New South Wales, Australia of more than 500,000 deliveries and showed significantly increased risks for OASIS with vacuum and forceps deliveries in both nulliparous and multiparous women, with forceps deliveries carrying the highest risk [7].

Studies from the Unites States showed that vacuum extractions and forceps deliveries in the USA are also associated with an increased risk for OASIS. However, in the study of Handa et al. use of the vacuum extraction carried a larger risk for OASIS than forceps delivery [2].

The more recent study from Landy et al. showed results that were comparable to the European studies for women delivering their first baby, but showed a higher risk with the use of vacuum extraction in multiparous women [6].

For a direct comparison between vacuum extraction and forceps delivery in randomised clinical trials with regard to their risk for the occurrence of OASIS, we can rely on the results of the most recent Cochrane review on this subject. This review shows that the risk for OASIS in forceps deliveries is almost 90 % higher than in vacuum extractions (risk ratio 1.89; 95 % CI 1.51–2.37) [8].

Thus, operative vaginal deliveries are associated with an increased risk for OASIS in comparison with spontaneous delivery. In this, forceps delivery most probably carries a higher risk than vacuum delivery. Therefore, if the obstetric situation permits use of either instrument, vacuum extraction should be the preferred.

Duration of the Second Stage of Labour

The association of the duration of the second stage of labour with the occurrence of OASIS can be expressed in different ways.

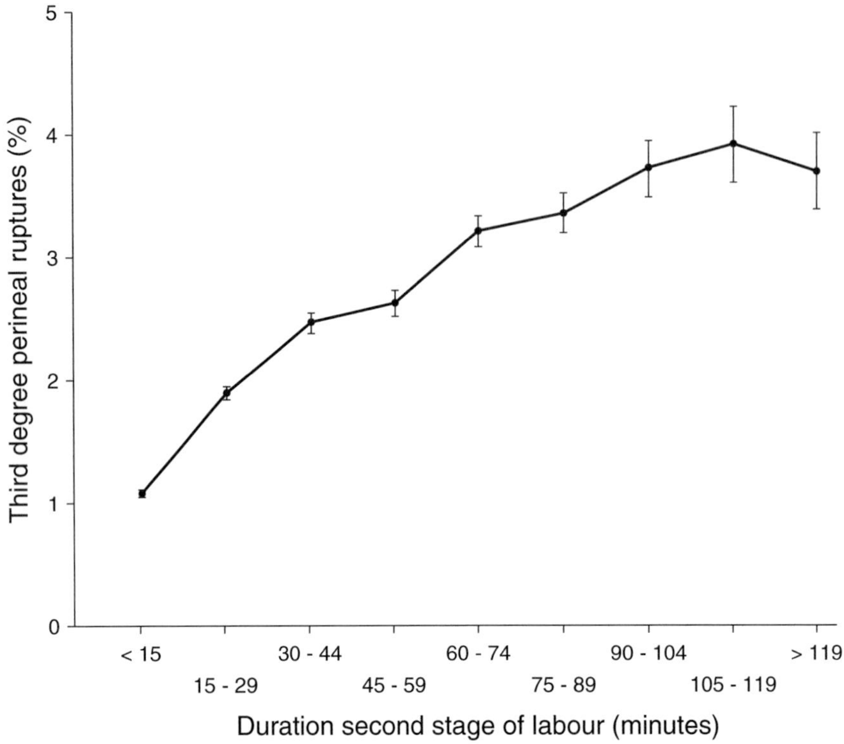

Fig. 4.2 Risk of third degree perineal ruptures per 15 min duration of second stage of labour (Reprinted from de Leeuw et al. [3] with permission from John Wiley and Sons, Inc.)

De Leeuw et al. showed an increase of the risk for OASIS of 12 % with every 15 min of pushing [3]. The actual rate of OASIS per 15 min duration of second stage is shown in Fig. 4.2.

These results were confirmed by the study of Räisänen et al. with an even stronger association [4]. In this study the risk of OASIS was doubled after more than 60 min of active pushing, compared to situations with an active second stage of less than 15 min in nulliparous women. In multiparous women the risk of OASIS showed a sevenfold increase with a second stage of more than 60 min.

Gottvall et al. expressed the association of the risk of OASIS with the length of second stage as a dichotomous variable. A second stage of more than 1 h was associated with a relative increase in risk for OASIS by 50 % [9].

The association of the length of second stage with the occurrence of OASIS needs to be handled with care for several reasons: Firstly, whether the use of upper time limits for the duration of second stage will lower the risk of anal sphincter damage in daily obstetric practice remains doubtful, as this will lead to an increase in operative vaginal deliveries which may carry an even larger burden for the anal sphincters; Secondly, some of the databases used for population studies do not discriminate between the second stage and the pushing phase; and finally, It is not always feasible to know the exact time when the second stage starts because this is reliant on when full cervical dilation was diagnosed rather than when it actually happened.

Abnormal Fetal Positions and Presentations

Persistent abnormal fetal position, e.g. occipitoposterior position is associated with a more difficult delivery. Indeed, it is more likely to be associated with a caesarean section or operative vaginal delivery because of an arrest during first or second stage of labour compared to an occipitoanterior position. If the baby is delivered vaginally, abnormal vertex positions appear to be independently associated with OASIS. Baumann et al. reported in their population based study containing more than 40,000 nulliparous women from the state of Schleswig–Holstein in Northern Germany, an almost doubled risk for OASIS in this situation [10]. This increased risk is in line with the results of other studies [3, 4].

This association can be explained by the fact that with occipitoposterior position the head of the baby passes the vaginal introitus deflexed (and hence with wider diameters), causing more stretching of the vaginal introitus.

In only one study the possible association of vaginal breech delivery with the risk of OASIS was addressed where no association was found [3].

Even though abnormal fetal head positions may increase the risk of OASIS, it explains only a small number of all OASIS and deliveries because of its low prevalence [3, 11]. It is therefore in the individual patient a factor to consider, but has only a small contribution to the total number of OASIS.

Maternal Age

Maternal age at delivery may be associated with the risk of OASIS because of changes in the elasticity of perineal tissue throughout life [4]. With advancing age connective tissue may become relatively less elastic which may lead to higher risk for OASIS during vaginal delivery.

Handa et al. showed in their study that women under the age of 18 had a smaller chance to sustain OASIS and that women older than 35 years had a larger chance to sustain OASIS, both compared to women between the age of 18 and 35 years [2]. This trend of risk increase with advancing age was also found by Baghestan et al. [5]

Studies that have made a subdivision between nulliparous and multiparous women showed conflicting results. Räisänen et al. showed that with advancing age the risk for OASIS was increased compared to the risk in nulliparous women younger than 20 years [4]. In the study of Landy et al. advancing age was associated with OASIS only in nulliparous women [6]. The results of the study of Ampt et al. showed that in multiparous women, advancing age was associated with the risk of

OASIS up to the age of 40. In nulliparous women this association was found only in women until the age of 30. After the age of 30 in nulliparous, and after the age of 40 in multiparous women, no further increase in risk for OASIS was found [7].

In conclusion, advancing age may be associated with an increasing risk of OASIS during vaginal delivery, but this association may differ between nulli- and multiparous women and is only of relative importance because of its relatively weak association.

Maternal Body Mass Index

Body mass index (BMI) is investigated in only few studies probably because weight and height are not routinely registered in all maternity registries.

A BMI between 20 and 25 is considered normal and the group of women with a BMI below 25 served as reference group in most studies that addressed this factor.

In the study of Hamilton from the USA defining high-risk risk clusters for OASIS, increasing BMI was negatively associated, although not strongly, with the risk of OASIS (OR 0.97; 95 % CI:0.95–0.99) [11].

Lindholm and Altman found in their study, describing more than 200,000 women who delivered in Sweden between 2003 and 2008, that increasing BMI was associated with a significant decrease in risk of OASIS [12]. Women with a BMI >35 had a 30 % lesser chance to develop OASIS compared to the reference group of women with a BMI <25. Landy et al. showed a significant negative association of BMI with the risk of OASIS only in nulliparous women with a BMI 30–34 compared with women with a BMI <25. In multiparous women no association was found in their study [6].

Explanations of the inverse relation of BMI with OASIS are speculative. Lindholm and Altman hypothesized that higher cholesterol levels in women with higher BMI may be protective to oxytocin overstimulation during the second stage of labour by modulation of oxytocin receptor efficacy in uterine smooth muscle.

Pain Relief During Delivery

Although epidural analgesia serves as the most widespread method of pain relief for women during the first stage of delivery in modern obstetrics, other methods are still in use in different countries e.g. nitrous oxide gas or pethidine.

The effect of epidural analgesia for pain relief on the risk of OASIS is still a matter of debate because of conflicting results in different studies from different countries.

In the study of Baumann et al. epidural analgesia was associated with a decrease of more than 30 % of the risk of OASIS without a subdivision for parity [10]. Landy et al. found a similar association of decreased risk for both nulliparous and multiparous women [6].

The population-based study from Baghestan et al. from Norway found no association of the use of epidural with the risk of OASIS [5].

The studies of Räisänen et al. and Ampt et al. confirmed this effect for nulliparous women only [4, 7]. In these studies the risk of OASIS appeared to be increased for multiparous women delivering with epidural analgesia.

Räisänen et al. have reported also on the effect of nitrous oxide gas on the risk of OASIS. In both nulliparous and multiparous women, the use of nitrous oxide gas was associated with a slightly decreased risk of OASIS [4].

The differences between the different studies mentioned may arise from differences in maternity-related practices between the different countries and may be caused by confounding through unknown factors that were not recorded in the various studies or registration systems used.

Induction of Labour and Oxytocin Use

The results in studies on effect of induction of labor and oxytocin on prevalence of OASIS are conflicting which again may be due to a difference in individual practices between the different studies. For instance, induction of labour may be used more often in women with intra-uterine growth retardation or post-term pregnancy in some countries or units compared to others.

Ampt et al. combined induction and augmentation of labour and found a decreased risk of OASIS in nulliparous women but no association in multiparous women [7].

Induction of labour was also addressed in the studies from Baghestan et al. and de Leeuw et al. [3, 5]. In both studies induction of labour was associated with an small increased risk of OASIS. In none of the studies a proper explanation for this association was given and given the conflicting results, this factor is probably a confounding factor associated with other obstetric factors. Induction of labour was not associated with OASIS in a large, population based study from Norway [11].

Previous Delivery with Sphincter Injury

As OASIS occurs predominantly in nulliparous women, the chances that these women will conceive and have to deliver again is reasonable. In the process of proper counselling, it is therefore important to know whether these women have an increased risk of recurrence.

Elfaghi et al. were the first to address this issue and found that a history of OASIS resulted in a more than fourfold increased risk in the subsequent delivery. This risk appeared to be related to the extent of OASIS in the first delivery, as the risk of recurrence was even higher after a fourth degree rupture in the first delivery [13].

This association was later confirmed by the studies from Baghestan et al. and Jangö et al. with comparable odds ratios [14, 15]. The latter study confirmed that the degree of OASIS in the first delivery was an independent risk factor for recurrence. The risk of recurrence was relatively 70 % higher after a 4th degree tear in the first delivery compared to a 3rd degree tear in the first delivery.

A possible explanation for the association of a history of OASIS with a higher risk of recurrence in the next delivery might be scarring of the perineum and anal sphincter muscles. Scar tissue may be more vulnerable to damage after stretch leading to a higher risk of recurrence of OASIS. The fact that OASIS in itself is an independent risk factor for recurrence is important in the counselling process of women and for the attending physician or midwife in the next delivery. In daily practice many women with a history of OASIS will be anxious to experience this type of trauma again.

Previous Delivery by Cesarean Section

Women who deliver vaginally after a prior caesarean section (CS) were considered to be the same as nulliparous women with regard to their risk for OASIS. However, this may be dependent on the reason leading to the CS in the first delivery.

Räisänen et al. found that the risk of OASIS in the delivery after a CS in the first delivery was 42 % higher compared to women who had delivered vaginally in their first pregnancy [16].

The risk of OASIS in the pregnancy after prior CS was compared to the risk for nulliparous women to sustain OASIS by Baghestan et al. in 2010. Women delivering vaginally after prior CS had a significantly higher risk than nulliparous women to sustain anal sphincter injury, a result that was confirmed by Räisänen et al. in 2013 and Hehir et al. in 2014 [16, 17].

So, a CS in the first pregnancy is most probably an independent risk factor for OASIS during the next vaginal delivery. As stated by Räisänen et al. this may be explained by the fact that a relative fetopelvic disproportion leading to CS in the first delivery may also predispose to OASIS in the subsequent delivery since 40 % of the increased incidence of OASIS risk could be explained by fetal birthweight.

Maternal Ethnicity

Studies on the association of maternal ethnicity are often flawed by unclear definitions of ethnicity and lack of consistency of different subdivisions with regard to one ethnic group between different studies.

In two studies from the American continent comparisons were made between "white" women and women with other ethnicities [2, 6]. Handa et al. found that Asian women were at a higher risk to sustain OASIS compared to white women, with Indian women having the highest risk. In this study black women had a significantly lower risk of OASIS, compared to white women. However, Landy et al. were unable to confirm the latter result. In their study, only Asian women or women of the Pacific Islands were at higher risk for OASIS compared to white women.

Two Scandinavian studies also addressed the possible association of ethnicity with the risk of OASIS [5, 18]. Both studies compared the risk of different ethnic groups with the risk of European or Swedish women.

In both studies, African and Asian women were at a higher risk of OASIS compared to European or Swedish women. However, in both studies no further subdivision within the groups of Asian and African women was made e.g. in both Scandinavian studies the African women were in fact almost entirely women from East-African countries like Somalia, Eritrea and Ethiopia. A large number of these women were infibulated and the de-infibulation, performed before delivery may not have been completely protective. Whether the calculated risk for OASIS for African women in these studies also applies to women from West-Africa remains doubtful.

Synthesis and Conclusions

Many maternal, fetal and labour-related factors are associated with the risk of sustaining OASIS during vaginal delivery. Unfortunately many of these factors are non-modifiable, i.e. parity, fetal birth weight and obstetric history. Indeed, in daily practice, the choice of the instrument used in operative vaginal delivery may be the only modifiable risk factor.

Of all factors, nulliparity and *type of* instrumental delivery are the most important, because they are the most commonly occurring factors and in this carry the largest risk.

Knowledge of risk factors for OASIS and awareness among supervising midwives and physicians of the presence of these factors is an important step in the prevention of OASIS.

But it is important to realise that the vast majority of OASIS occur in women with a priori relatively low risk. Up to this date it appears to be impossible to make a proper calculation of the risk of OASIS or predict the occurrence of OASIS in the individual patient [19]. This implies that it is important that during every delivery the supervising physician or midwife offers risk reducing interventions to every delivering woman. Interventions that will be explained in Chap 5.

References

1. Sultan AH. Obstetric perineal injury and anal incontinence. Clin Risk. 1999;5:193–6.
2. Handa VL, Danielsen BH, Gilbert WM. Obstetric anal sphincter lacerations. Obstet Gynecol. 2001;98:225–30.

3. de Leeuw JW, Struijk PC, Vierhout ME, Wallenburg HC. Risk factors for third degree perineal ruptures during delivery. BJOG. 2001;108:383–7.
4. Räisänen SH, Vehviläinen-Julkunen K, Gissler M, Heinonen S. Lateral episiotomy protects primiparous but not multiparous women from obstetric anal sphincter rupture. Acta Obstet Gynecol Scand. 2009;88:1365–72.
5. Baghestan E, Irgens LM, Børdahl PE, Rasmussen S. Trends in risk factors for obstetric anal sphincter injuries in Norway. Obstet Gynecol. 2010;116:25–34.
6. Landy HJ, Laughon SK, Bailit JL, Kominiarek MA, Gonzalez-Quintero VH, Ramirez M, et al. Characteristics associated with severe perineal and cervical lacerations during vaginal delivery. Obstet Gynecol. 2011;117:627–35.
7. Ampt AJ, Ford JB, Roberts CL, Morris JM. Trends in obstetric anal sphincter injuries and associated risk factors for vaginal singleton term births in New South Wales 2001–2009. Aust N Z J Obstet Gynaecol. 2013;53:9–16.
8. O'Mahony F, Hofmeyr GJ, Menon V. Choice of instruments for assisted vaginal delivery. Cochrane Database Syst Rev. 2010;11:Art. No.: CD005455. doi:10.1002/14651858.CD005455.pub2.
9. Gottvall K, Allebeck P, Ekéus C. Risk factors for anal sphincter tears: the importance of maternal position at birth. BJOG. 2007;114:1266–72.
10. Baumann P, Hammoud AO, McNeeley SG, DeRose E, Kudish B, Hendrix S. Factors associated with anal sphincter laceration in 40.923 primiparous women. Int Urogynecol J. 2007;18:985–90.
11. Laine K, Skjeldestad FE, Sandvik L, et al. Incidence of obstetric anal sphincter injuries after training to protect the perineum: cohort study. BMJ Open. 2012;2:e001649. doi: 10.1136/bmjopen-2012-001649. Hamilton EF, Smith S, Yang L, Warrick P, Ciampi A. Third- and fourth-degree perineal lacerations: defining high-risk clinical clusters. Am J Obstet Gynecol. 2011;204(4):309.e1–6.
12. Lindholm E, Altman D. Risk of obstetric anal sphincter lacerations among obese women. BJOG. 2013;120:1110–5.
13. Elfaghi I, Johansson-Ernste B, Rydhstroem H. Rupture of the sphincter ani: the recurrence rate in the second delivery. BJOG. 2004;111:1361–4.
14. Baghestan E, Irgens LM, Børdahl PE, Rasmussen S. Risk of recurrence and subsequent delivery after obstetric anal sphincter injuries. BJOG. 2012;119:62–9.
15. Jangö H, Langhoff-Roos J, Rosthøj S, Sakse A. Risk factors of recurrent anal sphincter ruptures: a population-based cohort study. BJOG. 2012;119(13):1640–7.
16. Räisänen S, Vehviläinen-Julkunen K, Cartwright R, Gissler M, Heinonen S. A prior cesarean section and incidence of obstetric anal sphincter injury. Int Urogynecol J. 2013;24:1331–9.
17. Hehir MP, Fitzpatrick M, Cassidy M, Murphy M, O'Herlihy C. Are women having a vaginal birth after a previous caesarean delivery at increased risk of anal sphincter injury? BJOG. 2014;121:1515–20.
18. Ekéus C, Nilsson E, Gottvall K. Increasing incidence of anal sphincter tears among primiparas in Sweden: a population-based register study. Acta Obstet Gynecol Scand. 2008;87:564–73.
19. RCOG Green-top Guideline No. 29: The Management of Third- and Fourth-Degree Perineal Tears. 2015

Chapter 5
Intrapartum Interventions and Risk of Perineal Trauma

Katariina Laine, Sari Räisänen, and Vladimir Kalis

Abstract Investigating interventions to reduce perineal trauma faces several challenges including the wide variation in clinical practice and inadequate documentation of the actual interventions adopted by the obstetrician or midwife, like manual perineal protection (MPP), hence limiting the feasibility of properly assessing such interventions retrospectively. Several clinical interventions to reduce risk of perineal trauma at birth have been advocated with varying degrees of efficacy. Antenatal perineal massage, performed by the pregnant woman herself, reduces the need of episiotomy during delivery, but has no effect on spontaneous lacerations on the perineum. Selective use of non-midline episiotomy is associated with a decreased prevalence of OASIS, especially in operative and first vaginal deliveries. Perineal warm compresses during crowning/second stage of labour reduced perineal trauma in general, however the effect on risk of OASIS was non-significant. MPP has been shown to be an effective intervention in reducing the risk of OASIS in several large non-randomised studies. It is important to recognise that these methods will probably have no real impact on incidence of perineal trauma when applied on ad hoc bases. However, the introduction of a standardised and structured management protocol at the time of birth that is uniformly adopted by the entire multiprofessional maternity staff has been shown to significantly reduce the occurrence of OASIS. Indeed, combining MPP with slowing the expulsion of the baby's head

K. Laine, MD, PhD (✉)
Department of Obstetrics, Oslo University Hospital, Ullevål, Norway
e-mail: kattiksen@yahoo.no

S. Räisänen
University of Helsinki, Helsinki, Finland
e-mail: shraisanen@gmail.com

V. Kalis
Department of Gynecology and Obstetrics, Charles University, Biomedical Center, Medical Faculty, Pilsen, Czech Republic
e-mail: KALISV@fnplzen.cz

K.M.K. Ismail (ed.), *Perineal Trauma at Childbirth*,
DOI 10.1007/978-3-319-14860-1_5

(using two hands) and simultaneously coaching the mother not to push has reduced the incidence of OASIS by 50–70 % in large population based observational studies.

Keywords Manual perineal protection • Perineal massage • Episiotomy • OASIS

Introduction

Several clinical interventions aiming to reduce risk of childbirth related perineal trauma have been introduced, such as antenatal perineal massage, controlling and slowing the expulsion of baby's head combined with manual perineal protection, coaching the mother during pushing, episiotomy, using warm compresses on perineum during second stage of labour, stretching perineum during labour, using oils or lubricants and use of different pushing techniques (by natural need, immediate or delayed start of pushing). Studying the effect of obstetrical interventions and events on perineal trauma is challenging for many reasons. Most interventions are used ad hoc based on the clinician's experience and perceived indication. Moreover, there is wide variation in risk profiles of women giving birth. Hence, high risk patients who might need several interventions are not comparable with low risk patients giving birth without interventions. Furthermore, the type of clinical intervention, technique of performing it and indications for its use differ between countries and delivery units, and also between individual birth attendants. Indeed, many decisions in obstetrics are taken acutely with short time for consideration, and it is usual that decisions are based on traditions and previous experiences. Randomised controlled trials would be the best method to investigate effect of a treatment, however, small sample size, lack of blinding often impair the quality of trials studying infrequent events in obstetrics. This chapter explores studies assessing the abovementioned perineal protection interventions and challenges in research methods to evaluate them.

Manual Perineal Protection (MPP)

MPP (also commonly known as manual perineal support or hands-on technique) may include using one hand on the baby's head to slow its expulsion or only supporting the perineum with one hand, but some clinicians would include use of both hands in a definition of MPP.

Evaluating the use and effectiveness of MPP in reducing perineal trauma is difficult to study for several reasons: International agreement for a standardised definition for MPP is lacking, and therefore understanding of which technique for perineal support is actually used in clinical practice is often unclear; MPP is rarely documented in individual patient records or medical birth registries limiting the ability to evaluate such techniques in large scale population-based studies.

MPP during the second stage of labour has been recommended in many old textbooks, Ritgen's maneuver probably being the most well-known method for perineal manipulation during delivery, several modifications of this maneuver are also described [1]. More recently, it has been widely debated whether performing perineal manipulation, or manual support, has any effect on perineal trauma. In a survey of midwives in the UK half of the participating midwives reported that they prefer "hands-off" delivering techniques, even in cases of a high risk woman with previous OASIS, or a nulliparous woman with a large baby [2]. So, it seems like the use of MPP has been abandoned, or at least is not considered as beneficial in terms of reducing perineal trauma by many midwives in the UK [2]. Interestingly, at the same time, OASIS rates has increased in many countries [3–10].

Several studies from Nordic countries conclude that the use of routine MPP reduces OASIS risk. In a study comparing two delivery units in Finland and Sweden, a fivefold difference in OASIS incidence was observed, with a lower risk in the Finnish unit where MPP is routinely used [11]. Several studies from Norway reported a notable reduction in the incidence of OASIS after implementing a universal multiprofessional training programme for MPP to their delivery suite staff. Indeed, these studies revealed a 40–70 % reduction in OASIS rate in six Norwegian hospitals [4, 12–15], from 4–5 % to 1–2 %. Following this, the Norwegian health authorities recommended a re-introduction of MPP methods, which led to notable, almost 50 %, reduction in OASIS incidence in the entire country [4] from 4.1 % in 2004 to 2.3 % in 2010. The OASIS incidence in Norway is now further reduced to 1.9 % in 2013 [16]. In an observational study from Sweden lacking perineal protection and difficulties in visualisation of the perineum were considered risk factors for OASIS. It is plausible that inability to properly visualise the perineum due to maternal birthing and/or the clinician's working positions hinder access to undertake MPP [17]. In a Danish study, perineal manipulation during second stage of delivery explored, and "easing the perineum" was associated with reduced risk of OASIS. However, no definition for "easing the perineum" was described in the paper [18].

Several Norwegian studies [4, 12–15], have described actions that in combination have contributed to the reduced OASIS rate:

- Improved manual delivering techniques using two hands:
  - Slowing the delivery of the baby's head with the one hand
  - Protecting the perineum with other hand
- Coaching the mother not to push when the baby's head is crowning
- Choosing a maternal birth position allowing the accoucheur to visualize the perineum
- Improved episiotomy technique avoiding midline cuts

Four randomized controlled trials on perineal manipulation are published, but none of the trials were designed to compare between hands-on with hands-off delivering technique on risk of perineal trauma. Only one of these trials had OASIS as primary outcome. In this Swedish study, women were randomized to either Ritgen's maneuver or "standard care", and hands-off delivering technique was not tested. Standard care was not described, defined or recorded in this study, and therefore it is unknown what was actually done during the delivery in the control group [19]. No difference in OASIS risk was observed between the groups, and both groups had a high occurrence of OASIS (6.3 % vs 5.3 %) compared to the Norwegian observational studies with reduced OASIS rates [4, 12–15, 19].

In the other three randomized controlled trials the outcomes were postpartum perineal pain reported by the patient, or perineal trauma in general, including all types of perineal injuries (degrees 1 to 4) and not only OASIS [20–22]. These three trials included all parity groups, thus mixing primiparous women with high risk for OASIS and parous women with much lower risk for OASIS [20–22]. The trials were underpowered to investigate OASIS, because the power calculations were not performed to assess OASIS rates, but much more frequent events such as perineal tears in general (all degrees from 1 to 4) or postpartum perineal pain.

McCandlish et al. (HOOP study) randomized 5471 women to either hands-on method (the midwife put pressure on baby's head with one hand and protected the perineum with other hand) or the hands-poised method, where the midwife kept hands "poised" to be able to put pressure on the head if needed, but not touching the perineum. Notable contamination of the hands-on method to the hands-poised group was observed, midwife compliance was lower in the hands-poised group (70 %) compared to hands-on group 95 %); reason to this difference was that midwives wanted to avoid too rapid expulsion of the head. Episiotomy use was not reported in the paper. There was no difference in the OASIS rates between the groups [20].

In the trial from Austria with 1076 women, the main outcome was perineal trauma in general and neonatal outcomes. Two different manual methods were compared, and hands-off was not tested. Either the midwife used both hands, one on the baby's head an one on the perineum, or was hands-poised, meaning the midwife having hands close to the perineum, ready to perform pressure on the baby's head to avoid extensive expulsion, but no touching the perineum. The shoulders were delivered by protecting the perineum with a two-hand method in both study arms. The study concludes that OASIS was more frequent in the hands-on group, but many weaknesses impair this trial. There were notable differences between the study groups; in the hands-on group the use of median episiotomy was frequent, 11.4 % compared to the hands-poised group with 6.5 % median episiotomies, which may have influence the outcome. Additionally, the hands-on group had lower parity than the hands-poised group, giving the study groups non-comparable risk profiles [21].

In the RCT by Albers et al. with 1211 women, the main outcome was perineal pain 24 h after birth, and three different perineal manipulations were tested: using warm compresses on the perineum, perineal massage with lubricant and not touching the perineum before crowning, thus hands-off perineum method was not tested. Few OASIS occurred, and no differences in OASIS incidence was observed between the groups (0.7 %, 1.2 % and 1.5 % respectively) [22]. These studies are often referred to, when hands-off delivering techniques are promoted, especially the HOOP study [20]. The authors' view is that this is an unfortunate misinterpretation, since none of the studies compared hands-on with hands-off delivering method. The HOOP-study did not conclude that "hands-off" delivery method would be preferable or recommended during delivery [23–25]. Additionally, the HOOP study concluded that the hands-on delivered women experienced less pain three days after delivery. A recent systematic review by Bulchandani et al. showed that, based on metanalysis of findings from several non-randomised studies, manual perineal protection significantly reduces the risk of OASIS [26].

Episiotomy

Episiotomy, one of the most common surgical procedures performed on women. It is a surgical cutting of the perineum to enlarge the vaginal opening for birth during the last part of the second stage of the labour [27–29] Sir Fielding Ould first described the episiotomy in 1742; it was initially reserved for women with difficult births such as prolonged second stage of birth or to expedite delivery in cases of maternal or fetal distress [30]. Later, at the end of the nineteenth century episiotomy was adopted worldwide and its routine use was concomitant with a shift from home to hospital births without strong scientific evidence of its effectiveness. Use of episiotomy was justified by the prevention of severe perineal tears, reduction of urine and fecal incontinence, better sexual function and being a straight, clean incision that is easier to repair and heals better than a spontaneous tear [31, 32]. To date, a large number of studies have explored birth outcomes between women giving birth with and without episiotomy.

Episiotomy Types

Several episiotomy types are currently in use as reviewed by Kalis et al.; the most well-known types are median, mediolateral and lateral episiotomies [33]. The median type of episiotomy begins in the posterior fourchette and runs along the midline through the central tendon of the perineal body, is preferred in the USA. The mediolateral type, defined as incision beginning in the midline and directed laterally and downwards away from the rectum, is the most frequently performed type of episiotomy in Europe [33, 34]. Lateral episiotomy begins laterally 1 cm or 2 cm from the midline and is directed downwards towards the ischial tuberosity.

Episiotomy and Risk of Perineal Trauma

One of the indications for the use of episiotomy is the prevention of severe perineal trauma. However, episiotomy by definition is a second-degree tear, because it cuts the superficial muscles of the perineum, and thus its actual aim is to prevent severe perineal trauma reaching anal sphincter. Previous observational studies have shown that an association between episiotomy and OASIS varies by episiotomy type. Several studies have demonstrated that the midline type of the procedure is associated with an increased risk of OASIS [35–39], whereas the association between mediolateral type of episiotomy and OASIS has been obscure; ranging from positive to negative association [7, 40–43]. Use of lateral episiotomy has been associated with a decreased prevalence of OASIS in nulliparous women and an increased prevalence of OASIS in multiparous women [44]. However, several limitations should be acknowledged when critically appraising previous studies assessing the association between episiotomy and OASIS. Firstly, the episiotomy techniques used have been poorly or not at all described in many of these studies. Secondly, differences in techniques of mediolateral episiotomy, especially angle of incision, have been demonstrated where a significant number of mediolateral episiotomies seem to be cut at an acute angle are, hence, more likely to have an effect as a median episiotomies [45–50]. It has been suggested that mediolateral episiotomy with an incision angle of less than 60° [51] or too acute an angel [52, 53] might be associated with an increased prevalence of OASIS compared with episiotomy with an incision angle of 60° or larger angle, respectively. It has also been suggested that the length of episiotomy cut is associated with a risk of OASIS where a longer cut is associated with a decreased risk of OASIS [15].

Results from previous RCTs comparing restrictive and routine use of episiotomy have suggested restrictive use of episiotomy (by indication only), since this practice appeared to have a number of benefits such as less severe perineal trauma, less suturing, and less healing complications compared with routine use of episiotomy. However, based on previous RCTs there is no evidence to suggest which of the non median episiotomy types (mediolateral or lateral) results in better outcomes. Furthermore, no consensus exists for episiotomy indications when restrictive episiotomy use is recommended.

Warm Compresses on the Perineum During Labour

Keeping warm compresses on the perineum during the second stage of labour has been studied as a method of reducing perineal trauma. Nevertheless, the temperature of the compresses, when to start or the duration of applying them is not described or defined in the literature. Both observational studies and RCTs have explored the effect of warm compresses on perineum during the second stage of labour and perineal trauma, and the results are conflicting. Two observational studies from the US showed a slightly protective effect of warm packs on perineum [54, 55]. However, in both of the studies the use of warm compresses was poorly defined, lacking details of timing and duration of the use.

A previous RCT (717 women) from Australia reported that using warm packs during the late second stage of labour reduced the risk of OASIS and maternal pain

[56], but as highlighted by the authors of the study, this trial was underpowered to study the risk of OASIS. Moreover, a substantial weakness in the study was that the standard care for the control group was not described. Another RCT (1211 women) from the US did not find any differences in perineal trauma among three study groups (warm compress to the perineum, massage with lubricant or no touching of the perineum until crowing of the infant's head) [22].

It is of note that if warm compresses are used on the perineum during the labour, too hot compresses may cause burn injury on the perineal skin and compresses with adequate temperature cool off quite soon (observation based on clinical experience).

Antenatal Perineal Massage

Antenatal perineal massage, or stretching the perineum, performed by the woman herself or her partner has been studied in some RCTs. A Cochrane review included four trials (2497 women) where women had performed perineal massage in 3–10 min, 3–7 days a week, 4–6 weeks before delivery. This review concluded that women practicing antenatal perineal massage at least four weeks before delivery were less likely to undergo episiotomy, but no statistically significant differences were demonstrated for the risk of perineal tears (1st, 2nd, 3rd or 4th degree tears). These results indicate that women should be made aware of perineal massage practices and its benefits [57].

Perineal Massage During Labour

Perineal massage or manual perineal stretching during the second stage of labour is frequently used in clinical practice, but few studies have explored the effect of perineal massage during labour on perineal trauma. Perineal massage with fingers performed by the midwife or obstetrician was assessed in an RCT of 1096 women, and no difference in perineal outcome was observed between the randomised groups [58]. Another smaller RCT involving 396 women showed similar results i.e. no difference in risk of perineal injuries between the groups randomised to receive massage or no massage during delivery [59]. Use of vaseline or oils during second stage massage of perineum has been described in small studies. A shortened second stage was observed, but no OASIS occurred in either arm of the RCT with 90 women in a study where use of vaseline was compared with no vaseline use during second stage of labour [60]. In an RCT of 164 women two different oils during second stage perineal massage were compared and, again, no difference in perineal in occurrence of OASIS or other tears were observed [61].

Maternal Birth Position

Birth positions during labour have been classified by several ways such as upright or recumbent positions. The existing studies have also classified delivery positions regarding to whether the delivering woman is in a lying position with her back on bed or upright as standing, kneeling, squatting or on all fours. The lying positions are classified regarding to the angle of her back to the bed being more or less than 45°, as semi-recumbent or lithotomy position, or lying on a lateral position. Maternal birth position is usually not recorded in patient records or birth registries and therefore large register studies are not available.

Several previous RCTs showed no effect of maternal birth position during the second stage on perineal trauma [62]. A Cochrane Review of five RCTs (879 women) compared upright (sitting, squatting, semi-recumbent 45° or more from the horizontal, kneeling and walking) or recumbent position (lithotomy position, lateral position, terndelenburg's position, knee-elbow and semi-recumbent less than 45° from the horizontal line) during the second stage of labour among women with epidural analgesia; no difference in perineal trauma requiring suturing between the two groups was found [62].

Another Cochrane Review of 22 RCTs (7280 women) among women without epidural analgesia did not find any differences in perineal trauma requiring suturing between women without epidural analgesia using upright (sitting, kneeling and squatting) or supine position (lateral, semi-recumbent with up to 30° from the horizontal, lithotomy and Trendelenburg) [63]. However, many methodological weaknesses such as small sample size and unclear registration and randomisation were acknowledged in studies included in these Cochrane reviews. Both reviews concluded that women should be allowed to make choices about their birth positions.

Furthermore, a previous retrospective observational study from Australia (2,891 women) found that lateral position was the most favourable and squatting the least favourable birth position if looking for prevalence of intact perineum [64]. A Swedish study revealed that standing position during the second stage of delivery was a risk factor for OASIS, probably because among the women in standing birth position it was difficult to perform manual perineal support or slow down the crowning of the head. The standing position may also allow the woman to push harder [65]. Another Swedish study showed that lacking visualization of perineum increased the risk of OASIS, indicating that a maternal birth position allowing the midwife to reach the perineum has positive effect on the perineal outcome [17].

In a delivering bed, a woman may have her feet on stirrups or on the bed. A randomised trial compared women delivered with feet in stirrups with women without stirrups during pushing in late second stage of delivery and no difference between the randomized groups and risk of OASIS was found [66].

Overall, it is of note that studies on effect of maternal birth position on maternal and fetal outcomes might be affected by several biases. Firstly, during the second stage, which might be quite long, most women prefer to try several birth positions, and the final position during the late active second stage might last only some minutes. Secondly, randomisation of birth position might be complicated due to maternal or fetal distress. A birth position, especially use of recumbent or supine position, might indicate a more complicated birth, because many obstetric interventions such as episiotomy and use of vacuum extraction or forceps are more likely to be performed in these positions due to practical reasons. Similarly, use of upright positions might be a mark of less complicated birth and indicates no need for interventions. For example, performing an episiotomy or vacuum extraction for women who is walking or standing is practically difficult. Alternative and upright positions are used on low-risk deliveries – and lying on back only when problems such as prolonged second stage complicate the delivery.

Pushing Methods During the Second Stage of Labour

Pushing methods can be classified based on when the pushing starts (early or delayed), whether the pushing is coached by the birth attendant or spontaneous or if Valsalva is used or not. When pushing on "commando" or by natural subjective need were compared, no difference in OASIS occurrence could be observed [67]. Coached pushing with closed glottis (Valsalva) during second stage of labour does not seem to affect the occurrence of OASIS [67]. However, in a randomised controlled trial a large number of participating women were not able to use the method they were randomized to, 15 % were not able to push with closed glottis, and 34 % of the women randomized to push spontaneously with open glottis pushed with closed glottis. Thus, contamination of the methods was a problem in both study arms, and may have influenced the results.

Challenges to Research Methods for Assessing Effect of Obstetric Interventions on Perineal Trauma

RCTs are the gold standard for evaluating effectiveness of medical interventions such as episiotomy and other obstetric interventions. In RCTs randomisation is used to create groups that on average should have an equal risk of outcome; independent variables such as mode of delivery, birth weight and parity should be exchangeable between exposed and unexposed women. Randomisation does not guarantee that exposed and unexposed will have the same risk of the outcome, especially if there are unknown or unmeasured risk factors (such as condition of the perineum or birth attendants' performance in this case) or an inadequate sample size is used. OASIS is a relatively rare outcome and associated with several risk factors (see Chap. 4), indicating that large sample sizes would be required in any RCT, even if the target population are women at high risk for this outcome. All previous RCTs have compared restrictive and routine use of episiotomy only (requiring an even larger

Table 5.1 RCTs of effect of episiotomy on OASIS

Study: authors, year, country	Episiotomy rate restrictive vs routine use %	Number per study arm	OASIS %	Population
Mediolateral episiotomy				
Murphy et al. 2008, Ireland [68]	All 52 vs 93	101 vs 99	10.9 vs 8.1	Primipara, operative vaginal deliveries
Dannecker et al. 2004, Germany [69]	41 vs 77	49 vs 60	4.1 vs 8.3	Nullipara
Eltorkey 1994, Saudi-Arabia [70]	53 vs 83	100 vs 100	0 vs 0	Nullipara
Belizan 1993, Argentina [71]	30 vs 83	778 vs 777	1.2 vs 1.5	Nullipara and primipara
House 1986, UK [72]	Nulli 32 vs 79	98 vs 67	Nullip 0 vs 4.2	Nullipara and multipara
	Multi 2 vs 48		Multip 0 vs 4.3	
Sleep 1984, UK [73]	10 vs 51	498 vs 502	0.8 vs 0.2	Nullipara and multipara
Harrison 1984, Ireland [74]	8 vs 89	89 vs 92	0 vs 5.6	Nullipara
Median episiotomy				
Rodriguez 2008, Colombia [75]	24 vs 100	222 vs 223	6.8 vs 14.3	Nullipara
Klein 1992, Canada [76]	Nulli 57 vs 81 Multi 31 vs 47	353 vs 350	Prim 13.3 vs 12.5 Multi 0	Nullipara and multipara
Comparison of median and mediolateral episiotomy				
Coats 1980, UK [38]		163 vs 244	11.6 vs 2.0 %	Nullipara

sample size), and have either used an inadequate sample size (Table 5.1) or had unexpected differences in independent variables between the groups suggesting selection bias [68]. Furthermore, inclusion criteria for these studies were poorly specified as both nulliparous and parous women with substantially different background risk of OASIS were included (Table 5.1).

Overall, it is of note that the results of previous RCTs did not study episiotomy versus no episiotomy, and thus the results do not indicate no use of episiotomy or that episiotomy itself, used by indication, is a harmful procedure. It is also noteworthy that current episiotomy use is already restrictive in most countries and episiotomy rates have been actually lower than the restrictive episiotomy use in many previous RCTs (Table 5.1).

In observational studies such as case-control, cohort and cross sectional studies adjustment is traditionally used to minimise between-group differences (exposed and unexposed), but despite this, a major source of bias is confounding by indication, especially in studies of comparative effectiveness [77–79]. Confounding by indication means that intervention is reserved for the patients with more severe disease or condition. In obstetrics almost all interventions are used by indication and women who get or do not get the specific intervention are different. For example, episiotomy is more likely to be performed to women who are at higher risk of OASIS such as women who are nulliparous, need operative vaginal delivery or give birth a large infant. In other words, an intervention (here episiotomy) is reserved to women with higher risk of OASIS, which also is an outcome of interest in this case. Thus, women giving birth with and without episiotomy are not exchangeable or comparable, and an association between outcome and exposure is more likely to be harmful [80, 81]. Similarly, other obstetric interventions such as oxytocin augmentation, operative vaginal delivery and pain relief are reserved for women with prolonged or otherwise complicated and more painful labour. Consequently, results of observational studies are likely to be biased by confounding indication, but also unmeasured factors (not adjusted in analyses), which are associated with a risk of outcome. In many observational studies source of data is a register or other administrative database, which compiles limited information. In case of episiotomy and OASIS, registers usually do not provide all important information such as on use of manual perineal protection, condition of perineum or birth attendants' attitudes towards an intervention.

References

1. Cunningham F, Leveno K, Bloom S, Hauth J, Rouse D, Spong C, editors. Williams Obstetrics. 23rd ed. McGraw-Hill Companies, USA. 2010.
2. Trochez R, Waterfield M, Freeman RM. Hands on or hands off the perineum: a survey of care of the perineum in labour (HOOPS). Int Urogynecol J. 2011;22(10):1279–85.
3. Laine K, Gissler M, Pirhonen J. Changing incidence of anal sphincter tears in four Nordic countries through the last decades. Eur J Obstet Gynecol Reprod Biol. 2009;146(1):71–5.
4. Laine K, Rotvold W, Staff AC. Are obstetric anal sphincter ruptures preventable?- Large and consistent rupture rate variations between the Nordic countries and between delivery units in Norway. Acta Obstet Gynecol Scand. 2012;92(1):94–100.
5. Räisänen S, Vehviläinen-Julkunen K, Gissler M, Heinonen S. The increased incidence of obstetric anal sphincter rupture–an emerging trend in Finland. Prev Med. 2009;49(6):535–40.
6. Ekeus C, Nilsson E, Gottvall K. Increasing incidence of anal sphincter tears among primiparas in Sweden: a population-based register study. Acta Obstet Gynecol Scand. 2008;87(5):564–73.
7. Baghestan E, Irgens LM, Bordahl PE, Rasmussen S. Trends in risk factors for obstetric anal sphincter injuries in Norway. Obstet Gynecol. 2010;116(1):25–34.
8. Gurol-Urganci I, Cromwell DA, Edozien LC, Mahmood TA, Adams EJ, Richmond DH, et al. Third- and fourth-degree perineal tears among primiparous women in England between 2000 and 2012: time trends and risk factors. BJOG. 2013;120(12):1516–25.
9. Tyagi V, Perera M, Guerrero K. Trends in obstetric anal sphincter injuries over 10 years. J Obstet Gynaecol. 2013;33(8):844–9.
10. Ismail SI, Puyk B. The rise of obstetric anal sphincter injuries (OASIS): 11-year trend analysis using patient episode database for Wales (PEDW) data. J Obstet Gynaecol. 2014;34:495–8.
11. Pirhonen JP, Grenman SE, Haadem K, Gudmundsson S, Lindqvist P, Siihola S, et al. Frequency of anal sphincter rupture at delivery in Sweden and Finland–result of difference in manual help to the baby's head. Acta Obstet Gynecol Scand. 1998;77(10):974–7.

12. Laine K, Pirhonen T, Rolland R, Pirhonen J. Decreasing the incidence of anal sphincter tears during delivery. Obstet Gynecol. 2008;111(5):1053–7.
13. Laine K, Skjeldestad FE, Sandvik L, Staff AC. Incidence of obstetric anal sphincter injuries after training to protect the perineum: cohort study. BMJ Open. 2012;2(5) doi:10.1136/bmjopen-2012-001649. Print 2012.
14. Hals E, Øian P, Pirhonen T, Gissler M, Hjelle S, Nilsen EB, et al. A multicenter interventional program to reduce the incidence of anal sphincter tears. Obstet Gynecol. 2010;116(4):901–8.
15. Stedenfeldt M, Oian P, Gissler M, Blix E, Pirhonen J. Risk factors for obstetric anal sphincter injury after a successful multicentre interventional programme. BJOG. 2014;121(1):83–91.
16. The Medical Birth Registry, MBR. The medical birth registry, Norwegian Institute of Public Health. Available at: www.mfr.no.
17. Samuelsson E, Ladfors L, Wennerholm UB, Gåreberg B, Nyberg K, Hagberg H. Anal sphincter tears: prospective study of obstetric risk factors. BJOG. 2000;107(7):926–31.
18. Parnell C, Langhoff-Roos J, Moller H. Conduct of labor and rupture of the sphincter ani. Acta Obstet Gynecol Scand. 2001;80(3):256–61.
19. Jönsson ER, Elfaghi I, Rydhström H, Herbst A. Modified Ritgen's maneuver for anal sphincter injury at delivery: a randomized controlled trial. Obstet Gynecol. 2008;112(2 Pt 1):212–7.
20. McCandlish R, Bowler U, van Asten H, Berridge G, Winter C, Sames L, et al. A randomised controlled trial of care of the perineum during second stage of normal labour. Br J Obstet Gynaecol. 1998;105(12):1262–72.
21. Mayerhofer K, Bodner-Adler B, Bodner K, Rabl M, Kaider A, Wagenbichler P, et al. Traditional care of the perineum during birth. A prospective, randomized, multicenter study of 1,076 women. J Reprod Med. 2002;47(6):477–82.
22. Albers LL, Sedler KD, Bedrick EJ, Teaf D, Peralta P. Midwifery care measures in the second stage of labor and reduction of genital tract trauma at birth: a randomized trial. J Midwifery Womens Health. 2005;50(5):365–72.
23. McCarthy R. Protecting the perineum; have we been duped by HOOP? Br J Midwifery. 2009;17(12):779.
24. Freeman RM. Can we prevent childbirth-related pelvic floor dysfunction? BJOG. 2013;120(2):137–40.
25. Aasheim V, Nilsen AB, Lukasse M, Reinar LM. Perineal techniques during the second stage of labour for reducing perineal trauma. Cochrane Database Syst Rev. 2011;12(12):CD006672.
26. Bulchandani S, Watts E, Sucharitha A, Yates D, Ismail KM. Manual perineal support at the time of childbirth: a systematic review and meta-analysis. BJOG. 2015;122(9):1157–65.
27. Thacker SB, Banta HD. Benefits and risks of episiotomy: an interpretative review of the English language literature, 1860–1980. Obstet Gynecol Surv. 1983;38(6):322–38.
28. Carroli G, Mignini L. Episiotomy for vaginal birth. Cochrane Database Syst Rev. 2009;1(1):CD000081.
29. Graham ID, Carroli G, Davies C, Medves JM. Episiotomy rates around the world: an update. Birth. 2005;32(3):219–23.
30. Ould F. Treatise of midwifery. Dublin: Nelson and Connor; 1742.
31. Cleary-Goldman J, Robinson JN. The role of episiotomy in current obstetric practice. Semin Perinatol. 2003;27(1):3–12.
32. Lede RL, Belizan JM, Carroli G. Is routine use of episiotomy justified? Am J Obstet Gynecol. 1996;174(5):1399–402.
33. Kalis V, Laine K, de Leeuw JW, Ismail KM, Tincello DG. Classification of episiotomy: towards a standardisation of terminology. BJOG. 2012;119(5):522–6.
34. Kalis V, Stepan Jr J, Horak M, Roztocil A, Kralickova M, Rokyta Z. Definitions of mediolateral episiotomy in Europe. Int J Gynaecol Obstet. 2008;100(2):188–9.
35. Fitzgerald MP, Weber AM, Howden N, Cundiff GW, Brown MB. Risk factors for anal sphincter tear during vaginal delivery. Obstet Gynecol. 2007;109(1):29–34.
36. Dandolu V, Chatwani A, Harmanli O, Floro C, Gaughan JP, Hernandez E. Risk factors for obstetrical anal sphincter lacerations. Int Urogynecol J Pelvic Floor Dysfunct. 2005;16(4):304–7.

37. Handa VL, Danielsen BH, Gilbert WM. Obstetric anal sphincter lacerations. Obstet Gynecol. 2001;98(2):225–30.
38. Coats PM, Chan KK, Wilkins M, Beard RJ. A comparison between midline and mediolateral episiotomies. Br J Obstet Gynaecol. 1980;87(5):408–12.
39. Shiono P, Klebanoff MA, Carey JC. Midline episiotomies: more harm than good? Obstet Gynecol. 1990;75(5):765–70.
40. Revicky V, Nirmal D, Mukhopadhyay S, Morris EP, Nieto JJ. Could a mediolateral episiotomy prevent obstetric anal sphincter injury? Eur J Obstet Gynecol Reprod Biol. 2010;150(2):142–6.
41. Andrews V, Sultan AH, Thakar R, Jones PW. Risk factors for obstetric anal sphincter injury: a prospective study. Birth. 2006;33(2):117–22.
42. Sheiner E, Levy A, Walfisch A, Hallak M, Mazor M. Third degree perineal tears in a university medical center where midline episiotomies are not performed. Arch Gynecol Obstet. 2005;271(4):307–10.
43. de Leeuw JW, de Wit C, Kuijken JP, Bruinse HW. Mediolateral episiotomy reduces the risk for anal sphincter injury during operative vaginal delivery. BJOG. 2008;115(1):104–8.
44. Räisänen SH, Vehviläinen-Julkunen K, Gissler M, Heinonen S. Lateral episiotomy protects primiparous but not multiparous women from obstetric anal sphincter rupture. Acta Obstet Gynecol Scand. 2009;88(12):1365–72.
45. Wong KW, Ravindran K, Thomas JM, Andrews V. Mediolateral episiotomy: are trained midwives and doctors approaching it from a different angle? Eur J Obstet Gynecol Reprod Biol. 2014;174:46–50.
46. Andrews V, Thakar R, Sultan AH, Jones PW. Are mediolateral episiotomies actually mediolateral? BJOG. 2005;112(8):1156–8.
47. Tincello DG, Williams A, Fowler GE, Adams EJ, Richmond DH, Alfirevic Z. Differences in episiotomy technique between midwives and doctors. BJOG. 2003;110(12):1041–4.
48. Grigoriadis T, Athanasiou S, Zisou A, Antsaklis A. Episiotomy and perineal repair practices among obstetricians in Greece. Int J Gynaecol Obstet. 2009;106(1):27–9.
49. Fodstad K, Staff AC, Laine K. Episiotomy preferences, indication, and classification – a survey among Nordic doctors. Acta Obstet Gynecol Scand. 2016;95(5):587–95.
50. Fodstad K, Laine K, Staff AC. Different episiotomy techniques, postpartum perineal pain, and blood loss: an observational study. Int Urogynecol J. 2013;24(5):865–72.
51. Kalis V, Landsmanova J, Bednarova B, Karbanova J, Laine K, Rokyta Z. Evaluation of the incision angle of mediolateral episiotomy at 60 degrees. Int J Gynaecol Obstet. 2011;112(3):220–4.
52. Eogan M, Daly L, O'Connell PR, O'Herlihy C. Does the angle of episiotomy affect the incidence of anal sphincter injury? BJOG. 2006;113(2):190–4.
53. Aytan H, Tapisiz OL, Tuncay G, Avsar FA. Severe perineal lacerations in nulliparous women and episiotomy type. Eur J Obstet Gynecol Reprod Biol. 2005;121(1):46–50.
54. Hastings-Tolsma M, Vincent D, Emeis C, Francisco T. Getting through birth in one piece: protecting the perineum. MCN Am J Matern Child Nurs. 2007;32(3):158–64.
55. Albers LL, Anderson D, Cragin L, Daniels SM, Hunter C, Sedler KD, et al. Factors related to perineal trauma in childbirth. J Nurse Midwifery. 1996;41(4):269–76.
56. Dahlen HG, Homer CS, Cooke M, Upton AM, Nunn R, Brodrick B. Perineal outcomes and maternal comfort related to the application of perineal warm packs in the second stage of labor: a randomized controlled trial. Birth. 2007;34(4):282–90.
57. Beckmann MM, Stock OM. Antenatal perineal massage for reducing perineal trauma. Cochrane Database Syst Rev. 2013;4:CD005123.
58. Stamp G, Kruzins G, Crowther C. Perineal massage in labour and prevention of perineal trauma: randomised controlled trial. BMJ. 2001;322(7297):1277–80.
59. Karacam Z, Ekmen H, Calisir H. The use of perineal massage in the second stage of labor and follow-up of postpartum perineal outcomes. Health Care Women Int. 2012;33(8):697–718.
60. Geranmayeh M, Rezaei Habibabadi Z, Fallahkish B, Farahani MA, Khakbazan Z, Mehran A. Reducing perineal trauma through perineal massage with vaseline in second stage of labor. Arch Gynecol Obstet. 2012;285(1):77–81.

61. Harlev A, Pariente G, Kessous R, Aricha-Tamir B, Weintraub AY, Eshkoli T, et al. Can we find the perfect oil to protect the perineum? A randomized-controlled double-blind trial. J Matern Fetal Neonatal Med. 2013;26(13):1328–31.
62. Kemp E, Kingswood CJ, Kibuka M, Thornton JG. Position in the second stage of labour for women with epidural anaesthesia. Cochrane Database Syst Rev. 2013;1:CD008070.
63. Gupta JK, Hofmeyr GJ, Shehmar M. Position in the second stage of labour for women without epidural anaesthesia. Cochrane Database Syst Rev. 2012;5:CD002006.
64. Shorten A, Donsante J, Shorten B. Birth position, accoucheur, and perineal outcomes: informing women about choices for vaginal birth. Birth. 2002;29(1):18–27.
65. Gåreberg B, Magnusson B, Sultan B, Wennerholm UB, Wennergren M, Hagberg H. Birth in standing position: a high frequency of third degree tears. Acta Obstet Gynecol Scand. 1994;73(8):630–3.
66. Corton MM, Lankford JC, Ames R, McIntire DD, Alexander JM, Leveno KJ. A randomized trial of birthing with and without stirrups. Am J Obstet Gynecol. 2012;207(2):133.e1–5.
67. Roberts CL, Torvaldsen S, Cameron CA, Olive E. Delayed versus early pushing in women with epidural analgesia: a systematic review and meta-analysis. BJOG. 2004;111(12):1333–40.
68. Murphy DJ, Macleod M, Bahl R, Goyder K, Howarth L, Strachan B. A randomised controlled trial of routine versus restrictive use of episiotomy at operative vaginal delivery: a multicentre pilot study. BJOG. 2008;115(13):1695–702. discussion 1702–3.
69. Dannecker C, Hillemanns P, Strauss A, Hasbargen U, Hepp H, Anthuber C. Episiotomy and perineal tears presumed to be imminent: randomized controlled trial. Acta Obstet Gynecol Scand. 2004;83(4):364–8.
70. Eltorkey MM, al Nuaim MA, Kurdi AM, Sabagh TO, Clarke F. Episiotomy, elective or selective: a report of a random allocation trial. J Obstet Gynaecol. 1994;14:317–20.
71. Argentine Episiotomy Trial Collaborative Group. Routine vs selective episiotomy: a randomised controlled trial. Lancet. 1993;342(8886–8887):1517–8.
72. House MJ, Cario G, Jones MH. Episiotomy of the perineum: a random controlled trial. J Obstet Gynaecol. 1986;7:107–10.
73. Sleep J, Grant A, Garcia J, Elbourne D, Spencer J, Chalmers I. West Berkshire perineal management trial. Br Med J (Clin Res Ed). 1984;289(6445):587–90.
74. Harrison RF, Brennan M, North PM, Reed JV, Wickham EA. Is routine episiotomy necessary? Br Med J (Clin Res Ed). 1984;288(6435):1971–5.
75. Rodriguez A, Arenas EA, Osorio AL, Mendez O, Zuleta JJ. Selective vs routine midline episiotomy for the prevention of third- or fourth-degree lacerations in nulliparous women. Am J Obstet Gynecol. 2008;198(3):285.e1–4.
76. Klein MC, Gauthier RJ, Jorgensen SH, Robbins JM, Kaczorowski J, Johnson B, et al. Does episiotomy prevent perineal trauma and pelvic floor relaxation? Online J Curr Clin Trials. 1992;Doc No 10.
77. Psaty BM, Siscovick DS. Minimizing bias due to confounding by indication in comparative effectiveness research: the importance of restriction. JAMA. 2010;304(8):897–8.
78. Kallen B. The problem of confounding in studies of the effect of maternal drug use on pregnancy outcome. Obstet Gynecol Int. 2012;2012:148616.
79. Boyko EJ. Observational research–opportunities and limitations. J Diabetes Complicat. 2013;27(6):642–8.
80. Räisänen S, Selander T, Cartwright R, Gissler M, Kramer MR, Laine K, et al. The association of episiotomy with obstetric anal sphincter injury–a population based matched cohort study. PLoS One. 2014;9(9):e107053.
81. Räisänen S, Cartwright R, Gissler M, Kramer MR, Laine K, Jouhki MR, et al. Changing associations of episiotomy and anal sphincter injury across risk strata: results of a population-based register study in Finland 2004–2011. BMJ Open. 2013;3(8):e003216-2013-003216.

Chapter 6
Assessment and Postnatal Management of Genital Tract Trauma

Teresa Arias and Debra Bick

Abstract The majority of women who give birth vaginally will sustain some form of genital tract trauma and around 70 % of these women will require suturing of their perineal trauma. Current recommendations for routine clinical care from the NICE intra-partum guideline are that the assessment of the vagina and perineum to identify extent of any trauma sustained should take place as soon as possible. Repair should be performed using a continuous suturing method using a fast absorbing suture material. It is also recommended that women are advised on signs and symptoms of wound infection, including pain, exudate from the wound or the wound gaping, and signs and symptoms of genital tract infection. This chapter aims to consider the extent to which genital tract trauma impacts on a woman's postnatal recovery and outlines key areas for consideration for clinicians during the 6–8 week postnatal period and beyond.

Keywords Perineal trauma • Postnatal • Assessment • Repair • Continuous • Infection • Sepsis • Midwifery • Maternity

Introduction

The majority of women who give birth vaginally will sustain some form of genital tract trauma. The type of trauma sustained can range from bruising of perineal tissues, a spontaneous vaginal tear, a deliberate surgical incision (episiotomy) or

T. Arias (✉) • D. Bick
Florence Nightingale Faculty of Nursing and Midwifery, King's College London, London, UK
e-mail: Teresa.1.arias@kcl.ac.uk; debra.bick@kcl.ac.uk

K.M.K. Ismail (ed.), *Perineal Trauma at Childbirth*,
DOI 10.1007/978-3-319-14860-1_6

obstetric anal sphincter injuries (OASIS). It has been reported that around 85 % of women sustain genital tract trauma during vaginal birth, with data from primary research studies suggesting that around 70 % of these women will require suturing of their perineal trauma [46]. Type of trauma is likely to differ by mode of vaginal birth. For example, of over 400,000 women who had spontaneous vaginal birth and 83,000 women who had an operative vaginal birth in England in 2012–2013, around 8 and 75 % had an episiotomy respectively [30]. The shorter and longer term consequences for maternal health are well documented in large observational studies [27, 44] and can include pain [27, 58], dyspareunia [2], urinary and faecal incontinence, psychosexual difficulties and impaired mother-infant bonding [3]. Perineal wound infection was recently reported as a main concern for UK women following a second degree tear or episiotomy [33]. It is therefore imperative that postnatal management of genital tract trauma is accorded high priority due to the potential impact on a woman's physical and psychological wellbeing, her ability to care for her new born infant, her personal relationships and plans for future pregnancy.

This chapter aims to consider the extent to which genital tract trauma impacts on a woman's postnatal recovery and outlines key areas for consideration for clinicians during the 6–8 week postnatal period and beyond. Recommendations for service delivery will also be considered. National Institute for Health and Care Excellence (NICE) guidance and quality standards for postnatal care [48, 49] are referred to where relevant, including recommended timing and content of care during the postnatal period.

Management of Genital Tract Trauma Immediately Following Birth

Current recommendations for routine clinical care from the NICE intra-partum guideline [50] are that the assessment of the vagina and perineum to identify extent of any trauma sustained should take place as soon as possible following spontaneous or instrumental vaginal birth to minimise blood loss and potential for infection. This should not interfere with mother-infant bonding unless the woman has bleeding which requires urgent attention [50]. A thorough assessment should be made by a skilled and experienced practitioner, usually the midwife or obstetrician, followed by full documentation of the wound severity, site and any necessary repair, with classification of genital tract trauma adhering to NICE guidance (2007; [50], Table 6.1).

NICE [50] recommendations for assessment and management of genital tract trauma include the importance of good communication with the woman to explain all procedures being undertaken and why; ensuring that the woman is in a comfortable position; that there is good lighting to provide the clinician with a clear view of the perineal area and genital structures; and that care is gentle and sensitive. The following should be adhered to as part of a systematic assessment of genital tract trauma and preparation to suture (if required) based on clinical judgement:

Table 6.1 Classification of genital tract trauma

First degree	Injury to skin only
	Injury to the perineum involving perineal muscles but not involving the anal sphincter
Second degree	Injury to the perineum involving the anal sphincter complex;
Third degree	3a<50 % of external anal sphincter (EAS) thickness torn;
	3b>50 % of EAS thickness torn;
	3c Internal anal sphincter (IAS) torn
Fourth degree	Injury to perineum involving the anal sphincter complex (EAS and/or IAS) and anal epithelium

- Confirmation by the woman that tested effective local or regional analgesia is in place
- Visual assessment of the extent of perineal trauma to include the structures involved, the apex of the injury and assessment of bleeding
- A rectal examination to assess whether there has been any damage to the external or internal anal sphincter if there is any suspicion that the perineal muscles are damaged [50]

Repair of genital tract trauma should not commence until the woman has effective analgesia. Women who sustain a first degree tear may not require their wound to be sutured unless the skin edges are not well opposed. Evidence to inform benefit of suturing or non-suturing of a second degree tear is inconclusive, with NICE [50] recommending that muscles should be sutured to promote healing, but if skin edges are well opposed, suturing of the perineal skin is not necessary.

There is robust evidence to inform suturing methods and materials to repair genital tract trauma. Use of continuous compared to interrupted suturing methods were found in a Cochrane systematic review to be associated with less short-term pain, less need for postpartum analgesia and less need for removal of suture material [37]. Data were included from 16 trials from eight countries and over 8,000 women. Another Cochrane review of suturing materials which included 18 trials and data on over 10,000 women found that use of catgut to repair perineal trauma was more likely to be associated with short-pain compared with synthetic suturing materials [38].

Despite NICE guidance [50] recommending use of continuous suturing methods to repair perineal trauma, a survey of UK midwives which asked about their perineal management practice found that only 6 % of 338 midwives who met study inclusion criteria used evidence based suturing methods [5], highlighting a substantial evidence to practice gap. The Perineal Assessment and Repair Longitudinal Study (PEARLS, [6, 33]), which aimed to improve uptake of evidence based assessment and repair of perineal trauma through quality improvement and introduction of facilitator led training found a significant increase in use of evidence based clinical management in the intervention sites compared with control sites. There was no difference in the primary outcome of maternal pain when walking or sitting within the previous 24 h as assessed at 10–12 days following birth. However, there were differences in some secondary outcomes. Women were less likely to experience perineal wound infection or need perineal sutures removed [33].

OASIS has been reported to occur in around 1–4 % of vaginal births [22]. A retrospective cohort study of singleton births in England during 2000–2012 reported a rise in the OASIS rate over successive years from 1.8 to 5.9 % [26]. Speculation about the increased rate centred on improved recognition by the attending clinician rather than changes in maternal or obstetric risk factors [26]. Nevertheless, controversy exists as to the cause of the perceived rise in OASIS. It is thought that accoucheur approaches to supporting the perineum and communicating with the woman during the second stage may contribute, although there is no robust evidence to support this and further research is needed (Ismail et al. 2015) [34].

Women who have sustained OASIS should be managed by an appropriately trained clinician for assessment and repair of their injury, given the potential range of postnatal morbidity women may experience if trauma is not appropriately repaired (for example, faecal incontinence), with potential implications on future mode of birth [39] and for litigation [47] if this trauma is not dealt with adequately. Risk factors for OASIS include midline episiotomy, operative vaginal delivery, infant birthweight >4 kg and occipito-posterior position at birth (Sultan et al. 2007) [56]. Particular attention should be paid to immediate postnatal perineal assessment of women who have any of these risk factors. The Royal College of Obstetrics and Gynaecology (RCOG) guidelines for management of third and fourth degree perineal tears [54] should be adhered to, although further evidence of most appropriate technique for primary repair of OASIS is required [22]. A Cochrane review of methods of repair for obstetric anal injury which included six trials and data on 588 women reported wide study heterogeneity [22]. There were no differences in outcomes of perineal pain, dyspareunia or flatus incontinence using an overlap or end to end repair of trauma, but there were statistically significant differences in incidence of faecal urgency and anal incontinence scores in favour of the overlap repair group [22]. Women who have OASIS will require appropriate postnatal care, which in the immediate period should include a prescription for broad-spectrum antibiotics and use of postpartum laxatives to reduce incidence of post-operative wound infection (RCOG 2015). Longer-term assessment of the repair should be planned as part of women's postnatal management.

As repair of genital tract trauma is a surgical intervention, swabs and suture materials used should be counted and recorded before and after the procedure. Retained vaginal swabs are a notifiable adverse incident [47] with potentially serious medical consequences, psychological harm and psychosexual difficulties associated with these incidents likely to persist beyond the immediate postnatal period [31]. With the woman's permission, a digital rectal examination should be performed following repair to a second degree tear or episiotomy to check that no suture material has been inserted accidentally through the rectal mucosa. The extent of trauma sustained, approaches to management and plans for pain relief should be accurately documented in the woman's maternity records and discussed with her prior to transfer to the postnatal ward. NICE [50] recommend that rectal non-absorbable anti-inflammatory drugs should be routinely offered after completing repair of first and second degree trauma, unless contraindicated.

Care in First 24 h Postnatally

The majority of women who sustain genital tract trauma will experience perineal pain, particularly within the first 24–48 h post-birth. This may not only cause distress and discomfort but could also impact on aspects of the woman's transition to motherhood. For some women, perineal pain may persist for weeks or even months following the birth [18, 42] with some women still reporting pain at 6 months post-birth [11, 27]. There is cumulative evidence that instrumental delivery, episiotomy and OASIS are associated with a prolonged recovery time and morbidity [44, 55].

Assessment of severity of postnatal perineal pain has been investigated using a variety of methods, including visual analogue scales [19, 44] and general pain scales such as the McGill Pain Questionnaire Short Form [10]. The impact of perineal pain on daily activities has been used as a primary study outcome in two UK trials of perineal assessment and repair [33, 36]. There is no validated assessment tool currently available specific to postpartum perineal pain [6] and knowledge and assessment of pain by most health professionals is likely to be poorly undertaken [41]. Although further research has been recommended to produce a specifically designed evaluation tool to measure both intensity and quality of the pain which is appropriate and easily understood by woman and clinician [57], it remains an evidence gap.

There are potential shorter and longer term consequences for maternal health and wellbeing if perineal pain is not appropriately managed. In one recent study, semi-structured interviews were undertaken in preparation for a randomized controlled trial of cooling treatments to relieve perineal pain; 215 women were interviewed within 72 h of a vaginal birth [20]. Findings showed that 90 % of women who sustained genital tract trauma experienced pain, mostly on walking or sitting, however a third experienced pain when feeding their baby and 41 % felt that their ability to care for their baby was affected.

Several options for pharmacological and non-pharmacological methods of relief of perineal pain are available; the effectiveness of some of these was evaluated in Cochrane reviews. Rectal analgesia using non-steroidal anti-inflammatory drugs (NSAIDs) was considered in a review by Hedayati et al. [32] which included three trials with data on 249 women, although only data from two trials could be included in the meta-analysis. Women who received analgesia through use of NSAIDs were less likely to report pain at 24 h following birth compared with placebo. Women in the NSAID suppositories group compared with women in the placebo group required less additional analgesia in the first 24 h after birth (RR 0.31, 95 % CI 0.17–0.54, 1 trial, 89 women) and this effect was still evident at 48 h postpartum (RR 0.63, 95 % CI 0.45–0.89, 1 trial, 89 women). Data on longer-term pain outcomes were not considered, nor were effects on other outcomes such as the mother – infant relationship, dyspareunia or daily activities.

Another Cochrane review considered use of single administration of paracetamol to relieve acute perineal pain [13]. Data were include from ten studies which described two dosages of paracetamol, five of which assessed 500–650 mg dosages of paracetamol and six studies which assessed 1000 mg dosages. Due to the age of some of the included studies, it was not possible to assess the risk of bias, meaning that caution should be applied to findings. More women experienced pain relief with paracetamol compared with placebo (average risk ratio (RR) 2.14, 95 % confidence interval (CI) 1.59–2.89, 10 studies, 1,279 women) and significantly fewer women required additional pain relief with paracetamol compared with placebo (RR 0.34, 95 % CI 0.21–0.55, eight studies, 1,132 women). Both 500–650 and 1,000 mg doses were effective in providing more pain relief than placebo. No studies considered secondary effects.

Local cooling agents are interventions which women can control and apply themselves. A Cochrane systematic review by East et al. [20], which considered outcomes of different cooling agents, applied to genital tract trauma found limited evidence of effectiveness. The review included ten RCTs with data on 1,825 women. Interventions compared included cold gel pads, cold/iced pads, ice packs, witch hazel, pulsed electromagnetic energy (PET), hydrocortisone foam, oral paracetamol or warm baths. Ice packs provided better pain relief at 24–72 h postnatally compared with no treatment (RR 0.61; 95 % CI 0.41–0.91; one study, n = 208). Differences detected in a composite outcome of perineal oedema and bruising and overall wound healing were noted in one small study, favouring cold gel pads (n = 37) compared with ice (n = 35, mean difference (MD) 0.63 on a scale of 0–15; 95 % CI 0.20–1.06) or no treatment (n = 39, MD −2.10; 95 % CI −3.80 to −0.40) 3–14 days postnatally. Women reported more pain (RR 5.60; 95 % CI 2.35–13.33; one study, 100 women) and used more additional analgesia (RR 4.00; 95 % CI 1.44–11.13; one study, 100 women) following use of ice packs compared with PET.

When considering which pain relief may be most appropriate for an individual woman, the following may be useful to consider in addition to the effectiveness of the proposed medication:

- Acceptability to the woman
- Medical history and contraindications (i.e. asthma, contraindicated with ibuprofen and diclofenac)
- Compatibility with breastfeeding
- Side effects such as nausea, constipation, drowsiness
- Interactions with other medication
- Woman's attitude to medication route (i.e. if rectal analgesia considered)

Concerns that postnatal perineal pain was often underestimated, was the driver for a quality improvement initiative from Australia aimed to reduce pain in the first 48 h postnatal [60]. Pre-intervention, a small postnatal survey of 18 women was completed to assess pain levels and investigate pain management therapies used within 48 h of giving birth. The survey findings showed that perineal pain impacted negatively on daily activities, following which a number of initiatives were introduced into postnatal care following multidisciplinary consultation, including a guideline on pain management, an educational booklet for women on what to expect of perineal healing and a proactive approach by midwives to offer women routine ice packs and analgesia [60]. All women who sustained perineal trauma were assessed for contraindications to medication and offered paracetamol and diclofenac in the first 48 h post birth. A follow up questionnaire was distributed to 18 women following revisions to care, and pain scores before and after change in policy compared. This showed a 33 % increase among women reporting use of pain relief post-intervention. As the surveys only included a small number of women, conclusions cannot be generalised (groups were not matched for parity or degree of perineal trauma), but findings indicate that women may be more likely to use analgesia if effective practice change is introduced [60].

In addition to ensuring women who have genital tract trauma are aware of pain relief options and involved with decisions as to what they would prefer to use, clinicians should also discuss women's concerns about the healing of their perineal wounds. In particular, women should be aware that they need to advise their midwife or GP if they notice any offensive odour, discomfort or other pain from their wound. The attending healthcare professional should offer to assess the wound in cases of women reporting pain or discomfort from their perineum [49]. Observation of the perineal area should be undertaken with good light, and the woman in a comfortable position to enable the whole perineal area to be observed.

Accurate documentation is important, with some units introducing specific proforma to record site of genital tract trauma. If problems with wound healing do subsequently occur, the healthcare team involved could be extensive, highlighting the importance of accurate recording, approaches to wound closure and postnatal management. Effective communication between the health professional and woman can also impact on maternal well-being and satisfaction [53]. Some health professionals may communicate embarrassment or discomfort in discussions with women regarding female genitalia and adopt ambiguous language [28, 59], which may cause confusion or deter a woman from seeking further information or raising sensitive health issues [8].

NICE [49] recommend that all women should be offered information during the first 24 h after giving birth on signs and symptoms of potentially life-threatening conditions. Women who have had genital tract trauma should be advised on signs and symptoms of wound infection, including pain, exudate from the wound or the wound gaping, and signs and symptoms of genital tract infection including fever, lower abdominal pain and chills. Women should be advised that if they experience any of these symptoms, they should be reported to a health professional, who should examine the perineal area to assess signs and symptoms of potential infection and if necessary, escalate care to a perineal specialist or obstetric team.

Care in First Week Postnatally

Routine Perineal Assessment

Around 60 % of women are discharged home from hospital within 24 h of the birth [30]. Due to the decline in routine midwifery community contacts [12], information for women on wound healing processes, how to care for the perineal wound and signs and symptoms of wound infection is even more important. The following may be useful to discuss with the woman [49]:

- The extent of genital tract trauma sustained and the location of the injury
- Importance of good perineal care including importance of hygiene, hand washing before and after changing protective pads and after going to the toilet
- Importance of a healthy diet
- Likely length of healing time
- Pain management methods
- Coping strategies relating to passing urine and stools
- Who to contact with concerns regarding perineal healing i.e. GP , midwife, local perineal care clinic

A leaflet written to provide women with information about perineal care including how to look after their wound, the importance of a healthy diet and signs and symptoms of infection was included in the PEARLS study intervention package [6]. There was a statistically significant difference in numbers of women reporting that they had received information on perineal wound care among the intervention group compared to women who received usual care [33]. Although evidence of the benefit of pelvic floor muscle exercises (PFME) on perineal wound healing is not currently available, PFME may be of benefit for future health. Gentle muscular contraction and relaxation of the pelvic floor muscles may support revascularisation of perineal tissues and enhance soft tissue healing, with more active PFME encouraged when women feel more comfortable given potential benefits for improving the function of the pelvic floor. A joint statement by the Royal College of Midwives and the Chartered Society of Physiotherapy provides clear guidance for clinicians to ensure that information on PFME is consistently offered during and after pregnancy and robust pathways established to respond to women at risk of pelvic floor dysfunction [25]. Refer to Chap. 9 for more detailed information about PFME and childbirth related pelvic floor dysfunction.

All women who sustain genital tract trauma should be asked at each postnatal contact about their experiences of perineal healing, with those who report any concerns (for example, pain, discomfort, stinging, dyspareunia) asked by the clinician if they would like their perineum assessed [49]. Evidence from several large studies of postnatal care have reported the need for clinicians to specifically ask women about their experiences of more common morbidity, such as perineal pain, urinary incontinence and fatigue. Much morbidity remains 'invisible' if care only focuses on a 'traditional' content of physical observation such as assessing uterine involution or vaginal blood loss, as women may be reluctant to voluntarily report other symptoms [43].

The examination of the perineum in the postpartum period [4] aims to:

- Detect inadequate perineal repair or breakdown of repair
- Assess the process of healing
- Detect signs of infection
- Exclude haematoma

Women should be encouraged to continue with analgesia to relieve perineal pain with any concerns about ongoing or worsening pain referred to their midwife or GP.

Wound Healing

Wound healing involves a complex series of overlapping processes that restore tissue and function of the damaged genital tract structures (Table 6.2).

Monitoring Wound Healing

Knowledge of healing processes is an important part of a clinician's skills and competencies to provide effective postnatal care. The woman also may benefit from some understanding of these phases which may alert her to notify a health professional if poor healing is suspected. The assessment of normal wound healing in addition to implementation of evidence based recommendations for wound and pain care management are important components of routine postnatal care. The three intentions of wound healing include:

- Primary intention: tissues are restored by approximation with sutures and without need for granulation
- Secondary intention: the unsutured or dehisced wound achieves closure by granulation tissue filling the 'gap' of the wound. Healing by secondary intention can result in the formation of scar tissue, which is thick and less able to stretch. This tissue lacks suppleness and may contribute to postnatal dyspareunia as penetration may cause friction around the scar tissue [29].
- Third intention: closure is not achievable initially due to oedema or infection. This wound may be left for exudate to drain or kept open by packing and then debrided a few days later before surgical closure attempted [7].

Table 6.2 Wound healing process

Haemostatsis: Immediate response to injury. Vasoconstriction and release of plasma proteins
Inflammation: Commences within hours of injury and lasts between 5 and 7 days. Vasodilation and increased permeability of the blood vessels causing stimulation of pain fibres and localised heat, swelling and redness. (The health professional should note that an exaggeration of these symptoms may indicate infection
Proliferation: New blood vessels form throughout the wound forming a capillary network. A scaffold like structure of collagen forms around these vessels. Proliferation commences from 2 to 4 days after the injury. Rapid reproduction of granulation tissue and the migration of epidermal cells over the viable tissues commences.*Epithelial cells cannot migrate over an open wound, as in an unsutured wound , therefore the wound needs to fill with granulation tissue before this can occur. Bruising may be noted
Remodelling: The superficial healing may appear to have taken place but the reorganizing and remodeling of collagen along the lines of mechanical stress may occur at different times within the same wound. Remodeling usually commences approximately 20 days after the injury and may take up to a year to complete. Longer for open wounds Tensile strength increases though is thought to achieve approximately 80 % of the original tissue. Scar gradually fades and flattens

The Following Factors May Impair Wound Healing [49]:

- Infection
- Obesity
- Smoking
- Poor nutrition
- Environmental factors (lack of privacy, access to washing facilities)
- Medical conditions (e.g. diabetes)
- Poor primary repair of the perineal wound
- Stress related conditions
- Lack of sleep and stress

Wound Infection

Evidence of risk factors associated with genital tract wound infection following birth is limited as data are not routinely collated and women are likely to be managed in a range of secondary and primary care settings. A small prospective audit of women who gave birth in one English NHS unit and who had sutured perineal trauma aimed to identify infection using markers including pain, wound dehiscence and purulent vaginal discharge [35]. Data were collected over a 3-month period. Of 341 women who were followed up to 21 days postnatal, 39 (11 %) had a perineal wound infection (defined using two markers of infection), while 16 women (5 %) had all three markers. Risk factors significantly associated with infection included prolonged rupture of membranes and instrumental delivery. Webb et al. [63] suggested that infection is suspected when there is excessive discoloured exudate (rather than normal yellow) or smells offensive, abscess, erythema, or cellulitis. In these cases, wound swabs should be taken to identify causative organisms and antibiotics started in line with local guidelines.

Given concerns about maternal mortality due to sepsis in the most recent confidential enquiry into maternal deaths in the UK [40], and as an infected perineal wound could be a source of systemic infection, the importance of high quality, safe perineal repair and ensuring women are aware of the need to wash their hands with soap and water before and after going to the toilet, changing their sanitary protection or when touching their perineal wound is clear. Daily bathing or showering and ensuring sanitary protection is changed regularly are important to keep the perineal area clean.

Signs and Symptoms of Perineal Wound Infection [49]

- Increase in pain
- Oedema
- Abscess formation
- Cellulitis

- Excessive of offensive discharge
- Feeling generally unwell
- Pyrexia
- Wound dehiscence

Wound Dehiscence

Perineal wound dehiscence (dehiscence refers to a breakdown of the wound area) may be partial or complete and can be a consequence of a perineal wound infection (Thorpe et al. 2008). Currently there is no standardised approach to the management of perineal wound dehiscence although a large proportion of these wounds are treated expectantly [16] and research into the management of dehisced wounds is limited. Some authors have recommended that early repair of the dehisced wound is important to maintain perineal integrity [1, 62]. A recent Cochrane systematic review comparing secondary suturing compared with non-suturing of dehisced wounds to evaluate the therapeutic effectiveness of these two approaches found inconclusive evidence. Only two small studies of poor methodological quality were included in the review, with data available on 52 women. The lack of high level evidence led the authors to recommend need for further trials. The PREVIEW feasibility and pilot trial study which is aiming to identify the best management strategy for dehisced perineal wounds, in terms of clinical effectiveness and women's preferences is currently underway and will report shortly [17].

Care from 2 to 6 Weeks Postnatal

Usually around 10–14 days postnatally the care of the woman is transferred from midwifery to health visitors' care. For many women, severity of pain from genital tract trauma should have reduced, although pain may not have dissipated completely with 20 % of women reported to still experience some perineal pain at 8 weeks postnatally [20]. Women should continue to use analgesia for pain relief as needed, with women referred to their GP if they continue to report severe or new onset perineal pain, and clinical assessment of the perineal area as appropriate. Women should be encouraged to continue to perform PFME.

Sexual Health and Well-Being

Advice and guidance on timing and resumption of sexual intercourse, possible dyspareunia and use of contraception should be offered within 3 weeks of giving birth as some women will recommence sexual intercourse before the end of the postnatal period NICE [49]. A recent prospective cohort study which recruited 1507 women from Australia investigated timing of resumption of vaginal sex and assessed associations with method of birth, perineal trauma and other obstetric and social factors [45]. Sexual activity was resumed earlier than vaginal sex. By 6 weeks postpartum, 53 % of women had resumed sexual activity and 41 % had attempted vaginal sex. By 8 weeks, 65 % had attempted vaginal sex, 78 % by 12 weeks and 94 % by 6 months. When compared with women who had spontaneous vaginal birth with an intact perineum, women who had a spontaneous vaginal birth with an episiotomy or sutured perineal tear were more likely not to have resumed vaginal sex by 6 weeks. Women who had an assisted vaginal birth or caesarean section had raised odds of delaying resumption of sex. The delay in resuming vaginal sex could be due to women wanting to ensure that they are 'back to normal' following their final 6–8 week examination.

Dyspareunia (difficult or painful sexual intercourse) is reported to be common after childbirth, although there is limited evidence. A survey of 796 primiparous women at 6 months postnatal found that 62 % experienced dyspareunia in first 3 months [2]. The survey included questions on sexual problems commencing before pregnancy to 6 months postnatal; 32 % of women had resumed intercourse by 6 weeks postnatal, 62 % by 8 weeks and 81 % by 3 months. Painful penetration and or pain during intercourse or with orgasm was experienced by 62 % of women at some time in the first 3 months after birth and 31 % still experienced the problem when questioned. Findings should be treated with some caution. The response rate to the survey was only 61 %, the time interval between experience and participating in the survey could have introduced recall bias and the sensitive nature of the survey may have resulted in fewer respondents. Nevertheless, findings indicate women's willingness to discuss sexual concerns not identified by clinicians within routine postnatal care.

Referral to a perineal clinic may be of benefit to women experiencing painful intercourse after childbirth although further research is required into when and how to identify problems, as well as effective management and referral pathways. Although dyspareunia is a physical symptom, a woman could have underlying psychological problems, which should also be explored if women express anxiety about resuming intercourse. Expectations of pain during intercourse could start a cycle that reduces sexual arousal [15].

Women Who Are Breastfeeding

Breastfeeding has been associated with delayed resumption of sexual intercourse, possibly due to lack of vaginal lubrication and hormonal changes [52]. The study by Mcdonald and Brown [45] reported earlier, found an association between breastfeeding and delay in resumption of intercourse after adjusting for other factors including tiredness, which suggests that lactation may make an independent contribution to timing of resumption of vaginal sex after giving birth. If women who are breastfeeding report discomfort during intercourse, a water-based lubricant may be advised to ease this.

Six Week Postnatal Check

For many women, routine postnatal care will conclude with an appointment with their GP at 6–8 weeks postnatally, which has formed part of routine NHS maternity care for several decades in the UK. However, evidence of the benefit of this contact is limited and the contribution the contact may play in promoting longer-term maternal health and effective use of healthcare resources is, indeed, unknown. Current guidance is that women should be asked at the appointment about their general health and well-being and recovery from the birth, including healing of genital tract trauma [49]. The appointment is also an opportunity to ask the woman about resumption of sexual intercourse and use of contraception, although evidence is needed to support how well this information is provided, and the training needs of the clinicians who provide the contact.

Care Beyond 6 Weeks: Role of Perineal Care Clinics

Given the physical and psychological morbidity associated with genital tract trauma, particularly following OASIS [61], follow up referral to a consultant gynaecologist or obstetrician at 6–12 weeks post injury is recommended ([54]. Many NHS units have established perineal clinics led by a multidisciplinary team, which can provide a consistent approach to care for women who require ongoing review. A dedicated clinic has the potential to offer women sensitive, evidence based care provided by experienced practitioners [61]. There is limited evidence available regarding the benefit of perineal clinics [9] although contacts are considered to provide opportunities to provide women with an explanation of the injury sustained [23] and early assessment and treatment of pelvic floor dysfunction [9]. The most common indications for referral have been reported as OASIS and symptoms of urinary and faecal incontinence [23, 51]. Other reasons for referral could include dyspareunia, wound infection or dehiscence and ongoing pain. Endoanal manometry and ultrasound may be available or require further referral pathways. The perineal clinic may also contribute to advancing clinical knowledge and expertise whilst providing comprehensive care [61]. The multi-disciplinary team involved in the perineal clinic or the perineal care service may vary and could include a consultant gynaecologist/obstetrician, women's health physiotherapist, specialist clinical midwife, colorectal specialist, radiologist, recto-anal physiologist, tissue viability specialist, continence nurse and psychosexual counsellor [24].

Conclusion

Despite the high prevalence of genital tract trauma sustained during vaginal birth, robust evidence to support immediate assessment and repair of trauma, which could minimise shorter-term maternal morbidity, is not universally implemented.

Longer-term perineal care continues to be a neglected aspect of postnatal care. Although concerns have been raised about higher rates of OASIS and the reasons for this, there are calls for careful consideration of evidence prior to recommending revisions to perineal management during birth [14]. Antenatal and intra-partum perineal management should not be considered in isolation from postnatal consequences which for some women can be significant. Genital tract trauma morbidity may take months or even years to resolve, an aspect of maternal health that has been 'invisible' in terms of how care is planned and provided. Safe, high quality maternity care impacts on the woman's life-long health and it is imperative that it is managed as such.

Key Points

- Genital tract trauma is a common outcome of vaginal birth. It results in widespread postpartum morbidity with shorter and longer term implications for women's health
- Perineal pain is underreported by women. Health professionals should ask women at each postnatal contact about their experiences of pain and ensure pain requirement needs are met
- If women have any concerns about their perineum, the clinician should offer to examine the perineal area to check that healing is taking place as expected, with appropriate and timely referral if symptoms and signs of infection or dehiscence of the wound are identified
- Pharmacological and non-pharmacological approaches may reduce the woman's experience of pain and aid resumption of daily activities, including her ability to care for the baby
- All clinicians involved in childbirth should be competent in evidence based perineal assessment and repair, with access to regular training to update and revise perineal management skills
- Regular clinical audit against agreed standards for postnatal perineal management and health outcomes should be implemented in all maternity settings, which includes follow up of women to at least 42 days post-birth
- All interventions, including perineal management during and immediately following birth, should be evidence based
- Further research is needed into the management of perineal wound infection, role of perineal care clinics and sexual health postnatally

References

1. American College of Obstetrics and Gynecology. ACOG practice bulletin no. 71: episiotomy. Obstet Gynecol. 2006;107(4):957–62.
2. Barrett G, Pendry E, Peacock J, Victor C, Thakar R, Manyonda I. Women's sexual health after childbirth. Br J Obstet Gynaecol. 2000;107(2):186–95.
3. Bick D, MacArthur C, Winter H. Postnatal care: guidelines and evidence for management. London: Churchill Livingstone; 2008.

4. Bick D. Postpartum management of the perineum. Br J Midwifery. 2009;17(9):571–7.
5. Bick DE, Ismail KM, Macdonald S, Thomas P, Tohill S, Kettle C. How good are we at implementing evidence to support the management of birth related perineal trauma? A UK wide survey of midwifery practice. BMC Pregnancy Childbirth. 2012;12:57.
6. Bick DE, Kettle C, Macdonald S, Thomas PW, Hills RK, Ismail KI. The PEARLS study: enhancing immediate and longer-term assessment and management of perineal trauma: a matched pair cluster trial. BMC Pregnancy Childbirth. 2010;10:10.
7. Boyle M. Wound healing in midwifery. Oxford: Radcliffe Publishing; 2006.
8. Braun V, Wilkinson S. Socio-cultural representations of the vagina. J Reprod Infant Psychol. 2000;19(1):17–32.
9. Brincat C, Crosby E, McLeod A. Experiences during the first four years of a postpartum perineal clinic in the USA. Int J Gynaecol Obstet. 2015;128;1:68–71.
10. Briscoe L, Lavender T, O'Brien E, Campbell M, McGowan L. A mixed methods study to explore women and clinician's response to pain associated with suturing second degree perineal tears and episiotomies [PRAISE]. Midwifery. 2015;pii: S0266–6138(15)00005–4. doi:10.1016/j.midw.2014.12.010. [Epub ahead of print].
11. Brown S, Lumley J. Maternal health after childbirth: results of an Australian population based survey. Br J Obstet Gynaecol. 1998;105:156–61.
12. Care Quality Commission. National findings from the 2013 survey of women's experiences of maternity care. 2013. http://www.cqc.org.uk/sites/default/files/documents/maternity_report_for_publication.pdf. Accessed 08/03/2015.
13. Chou D, Abalos E, Gyte GML, Gülmezoglu AM. Paracetamol/acetaminophen (single administration) for perineal pain in the early postpartum period. Cochrane Database Syst Rev. 2013, Issue 1. Art. No. CD008407. doi:10.1002/14651858.CD008407.pub2.
14. Dahlen HG, Priddis H, Thornton C. Severe perineal trauma is rising, but let us not overreact. Midwifery. 2015;31(1):1–8. doi:10.1016/j.midw.2014.09.004. Epub 2014 Sep 18.
15. De Judicibus MA, McCabe MP. Psychological factors and the sexuality of pregnant and postpartum women. Journal of Sex Res. 2002;39(2):94–103.
16. Dudley LM, Kettle C, Ismail KMK. Secondary suturing compared to non-suturing for broken down perineal wounds following childbirth. Cochrane Database Syst Rev. 2013;Issue 9. Art. No.: CD008977. doi:10.1002/14651858.CD008977.pub2.
17. Dudley L, Kettle C, Carter P, Thomas P, Ismail K. Perineal resuturing versus expectant management following vaginal delivery complicated by a dehisced wound (PREVIEW): protocol for a pilot and feasibility randomised controlled trial 2013b. BMJ Open 2012;2:e001458 doi:10.1136/bmjopen-2012-001458.
18. East C, Forster D, Nagle C, et al. Women's experiences of perineal pain following childbirth. J Paediatr Child Health. 2009;45(Issue Supplement s1):A10–71. Territory, Australia.
19. East C, Sherburn M, Nagle C, Said J, Forster D. Perineal pain following childbirth: prevalence, effects on postnatal recovery and analgesia usage. Midwifery. 2012;28:93–7.
20. East CE, Begg L, Henshall NE, Marchant PR, Wallace K. Local cooling for relieving pain from perineal trauma sustained during childbirth. Cochrane Database Syst Rev. 2012;Issue 5. Art. No.: CD006304. doi:10.1002/14651858.CD006304.pub3.
21. Fenner DE, Genberg B, Brahma P, Marek L, DeLancey JO. Fecal and urinary incontinence after vaginal delivery with anal sphincter disruption in an obstetrics unit in the United States. Am J Obstet Gynecol. 2003;189(6):1543–9.
22. Fernando RJ, Sultan AH, Kettle C, Thakar R. Methods of repair for obstetric anal sphincter injury. Cochrane Database Syst Rev. 2013; Issue 12. Art. No.: CD002866. doi:10.1002/14651858.CD002866.pub3.
23. Fitzpatrick M, Cassidy M. Experience with an obstetric perineal clinic. Eur J Obstet Gynecol. 2002;100:199–203.
24. Fowler G, Williams A, Murphy G, et al. How to set up a perineal clinic. Obstet Gynaecol. 2009;11(2):129–32.
25. Gerrard J, ten Hove R. RCM/CSP joint statement on pelvic floor muscle exercise. Improving health outcomes for women following pregnancy and birth. London: CSP, RCM; 2013.

26. Gurol-Urganci I, Cromwell DA, Edozien LC, Mahmood TA, Adams EJ, Richmond DH, Templeton A, van der Meulen JH. Third- and fourth-degree perineal tears among primiparous women in England between 2000 and 2012: time trends and risk factors. Br J Obstet Gynaecol. 2013;120(12):1516–25.
27. Glazener CMA, Abdalla M, Stroud P, et al. Postnatal maternal morbidity: extent, causes, prevention and treatment. Br J Obstet Gynaecol. 1995;102(4):282–7.
28. Gott M, Galena E, Hinchliff S, Elford H. "Opening a can of Worms": GP and practice nurse barriers to talking about sexual health in primary care. Fam Pract. 2004;21(5):528–36.
29. Hay-Smith EJC, Glazener CMA. Persistent postnatal perineal pain and dyspareunia: A review of physical pathology and treatment. Crit Rev Phys Rehab Med. 1999;11(2):111–37.
30. Health and Social Care Information Centre. NHS maternity statistics – England 2012–2013. 2014. http://www.hscic.gov.uk/catalogue/PUB12744. Accessed 08/03/2015.
31. Healy P. Retained vaginal swabs: review of an adverse event in obstetrics through closed claims analysis. Br J Midwifery. 2012;20(9):666–9.
32. Hedayati H, Parsons J, Crowther CA. Rectal analgesia for pain from perineal trauma following childbirth. Cochrane Database Syst Rev. 2003;Issue 3. Art. No.: CD003931. doi:10.1002/14651858.CD003931.
33. Ismail KMK, Kettle C, Macdonald SE, Tohill S, Thomas P, Bick D. Perineal assessment and repair longitudinal study (PEARLS): a matched-pair cluster randomized trial. BMC Medicine. 2013;11:209. 23 Sept.
34. Ismail K, Paschetta E, Papoutsis D, Freeman RM. Perineal support and risk of obstetric anal sphincter injuries: a Delphi survey. Acta Obstetricia et Gynecologica Scandinavica 2015;94:165–74.
35. Johnson A, Thakar R, Sultan AH. Obstetric perineal wound infection: is there underreporting? Br J Nurs. 2012;21(5):S28–30. S32-5.
36. Kettle C, Hills RK, Jones P, Darby L, Gray R, Johanson R. Continuous versus interrupted perineal repair with standard or rapidly absorbed sutures after spontaneous vaginal birth: a randomised controlled trial. Lancet. 2002;359(9325):2217–23.
37. Kettle C, Dowswell T, Ismail KMK. Continuous and interrupted suturing techniques for repair of episiotomy or second-degree tears. Cochrane Database Syst Rev. 2012;Issue 11. Art. No.: CD000947. doi:10.1002/14651858.CD000947.pub3.
38. Kettle C, Dowswell T, Ismail KMK. Absorbable suture materials for primary repair of episiotomy and second degree tears. Cochrane Database Syst Rev. 2010;Issue 6. Art. No.: CD000006. doi:10.1002/14651858.CD000006.pub2.
39. Kettle C & Frohlich J. Perineal care. Best practice points. BMJ Clin Evid. 2015;03:1401:1–23.
40. Knight M, Kenyon S, Brocklehurst P, Neilson J, Shakespeare J, Kurinczuk JJ (Eds.) on behalf of MBRRACE-UK. Saving Lives, Improving Mothers' Care – Lessons learned to inform future maternity care from the UK and Ireland Confidential Enquiries into Maternal Deaths and Morbidity 2009–12. Oxford: National Perinatal Epidemiology Unit, University of Oxford 2014.
41. Kubecka KE, Simon JM, Boettcher JH. Pain management knowledge of hospital-based nurses in a rural Appalachian area. J Adv Nurs. 1996;23(5):861–7.
42. Leeman L, Fullilove AM, Borders N, Manocchio R, Albers LL, Rogers RG. Postpartum perineal pain in a low episiotomy setting: association with severity of genital trauma, labor care, and birth variables. Birth. 2009;36:283–8.
43. MacArthur C, Winter HR, Bick DE, et al. Redesigning postnatal care; a randomised controlled trial of protocol based, midwifery led care focused on individual women's physical and psychological health needs. NHS R and D, NCC HTA; 2003.
44. Macarthur AJ, Macarthur C. Incidence, severity, and determinants of perineal pain after vaginal delivery: a prospective cohort study. Obstet. Gynecol. 2004;191(4):1199–1204.
45. McDonald EA, Brown SJ. Does method of birth make a difference to when women resume sex after childbirth? Br J Obstet Gynaecol. 2013;120(7):823–30.
46. McCandlish R, Bowler U, van Asten H, et al. A randomised controlled trial of care of the perineum during second stage of normal labour. Br J Obstet Gynaecol. 1998;105(12):1262–72.

47. NHS Litigation Authority. Ten years of maternity claims: an analysis of NHSLA data – Oct 2012. 2012. http://www.nhsla.com/Safety/Documents/Perineal%20Trauma%20-%2013.pdf.
48. National Institute for Health and Care Excellence. Postnatal care. NICE quality standard QS37. 2013.
49. National Institute for Health and Care Excellence. Routine postnatal care of women and their babies. CG37. 2014.
50. National Institute for Health and Care Excellence. Intrapartum care: care of healthy women and their babies during childbirth. CG 190. 2014.
51. Pretlove S, Thompson PJ, Tooz–Hobson PM, Radley S. The first 18 months of a new perineal clinic. J Obstet Gynaecol. 2004;24(4):399–402.
52. Radestad I, Olsson A, Nissen E, Rubertsson C. Tears in the vagina, perineum, sphincter ani, and rectum and first sexual intercourse after childbirth: a nationwide follow-up. Birth. 2008;35:98–106.
53. Rowe RE, Garcia J, MacFarlane AJ, Davidson L. Improving communication between health professionals and women in maternity care: a structured review. Health Expect. 2002;5(p):63–83.
54. Royal College of Obstetricians and Gynaecologists. Third- and Fourth-degree Perineal Tears, Management (green-top guideline No. 29). 2015.
55. Signorello LB, Harlow BL, Chekos AK, Repke JT. Postpartum sexual functioning and its relationship to perineal trauma: a retrospective cohort study of primiparous women. Obstet Gynecol. 2001;184(5):881–90.
56. Sultan AH, Thakar R. Third and Fourth degree perineal tears. In: Sultan AH, Thakar R, Fenner DE editors. Chapter 4 Perineal and anal sphincter trauma. Diagnosis and clinical management. London: Springer-Verlag; 2007.
57. Steen M. Care and consequences of perineal trauma. Br J Midwifery. 2010;18(11(710)):712–5.
58. Steen M, Marchant P. Ice Packs and Cooling Gel Pads versus no localised treatment for relief of perineal pain: a Randomised controlled trial. Evidenced Based Midwifery 2007;5(1): 16–22.
59. Stewart M. 'I'm just going to wash you down': sanitizing the vaginal examination. J Adv Nurs. 2004;51(6):587–94.
60. Swain J, Dahlen H. Putting evidence into practice: A quality activity of proactive pain relief for postpartum perineal pain. Women and Birth 2012;26:65–70.
61. Thakar R, Sultan A. Postpartum problems and the role of the perineal clinic (chapter 6). In: Sultan A, Thakar R, Fenner D, editors. Perineal and anal sphincter trauma. London: Springer; 2007.
62. Uygur D, Yesildaglar N, Kis S, Sipahi T. Early repair of episiotomy dehiscence. Aust N Z J Obstet Gynaecol. 2004;44(3):244 6.
63. Webb S, Sherburn M, Ismail KMK. Managing perineal trauma after childbirth. Br Med J. 2014;349:g6829. doi:10.1136/bmj.g6829.

Chapter 7
The Role of Imaging in Assessing Perineal Trauma

Xavier Fritel, Anne-Cécile Pizzoferrato, Vincent Letouzey, Guillaume Legendre, Renaud de Tayrac, Katharina Jundt, and Arnaud Fauconnier

Abstract Pelvic floor disorders in women are highly prevalent affecting about a quarter of women with 10–20 % likely to have a surgical intervention for this pathology. A large proportion of pelvic floor disorders are related to perineal or pelvic floor trauma.

The purpose of this chapter is to appraise modern imaging techniques for the pelvic floor, discussing their strengths and limitations, and to suggest management strategies designed to effectively utilise imaging use in everyday practice.

Dynamic MRI provides an overall qualitative assessment of the pelvic floor and pelvic organ prolapse (POP). It achieves excellent differentiation of the type of prolapse in complex lesions. However, MRI staging is limited in everyday practice because it poorly correlates to the clinical examination. In order to avoid overtreatment a new MRI classification ensuring closer correlation with prolapse symptoms

X. Fritel (✉)
Service de Gynécologie-Obstétrique et Médecine de la Reproduction, Université de Poitiers, Faculté de Médecine et Pharmacie, INSERM CIC1402, CHU de Poitiers, Poitiers 86000, France
e-mail: xavier.fritel@univ-poitiers.fr

A.-C. Pizzoferrato
Service de Gynécologie-Obstétrique, CHU de Caen, Caen, France

V. Letouzey • R. de Tayrac
Service de Gynécologie-Obstétrique, CHU Carémeau, Nîmes, France

G. Legendre
Fédération de Gynécologie-Obstétrique, CHU d'Angers, Angers, France

K. Jundt
Department of Gynaecology and Obstetrics, University of Munich, Munich, Germany

A. Fauconnier
Service de Gynécologie-Obstétrique, CHU de Caen, Caen, France
Pr Arnaud Fauconnier, PU-PH, Service de Gynécologie & Obstétrique, CHI Poissy-St-Germain, Université Versailles Saint-Quentin, Versailles, France

K.M.K. Ismail (ed.), *Perineal Trauma at Childbirth*,
DOI 10.1007/978-3-319-14860-1_7

is clearly necessary. The main contribution of ultrasound consists in the study of pelvic-perineal meshes and urethral mobility assessment. Although endoanal ultrasound remains the gold standard for exploration of anal sphincter injuries, 3D perineal ultrasound can highlight atrophy or rupture of the anal sphincter while being much less invasive for patients.

Currently available studies have a low level convincing evidence for the usefulness of imaging in surgical management of urinary incontinence or POP. Nevertheless, the most interesting potential field of application for future management may reside in accuracy of detection of levator ani muscle avulsion as a predictor of risk of prolapse and surgical repair failure.

Keywords Perineal trauma • Oasis • Imaging • Ultrasound • MRI • 3D scan • Endoanal scan

Introduction

Pelvic floor disorders (PFD) in women are highly prevalent: about a quarter of women are affected by this pathology and 10–20 % are likely to have surgery for this problem [1, 2]. A large proportion of PFDs are related to perineal or pelvic floor trauma. In the United States, approximately 200,000 surgical interventions are carried out each year because of pelvic organ prolapse [3]. In France, about 42,000 cervicocystopexies are performed per annum [4]. PFDs seriously deteriorate the woman's quality of life with a wide variety of symptoms including chronic pelvic pain, urinary or anal incontinence, pelvic organ prolapse, constipation and anism. Recurrences or failures following surgical interventions are frequent with nearly 30 % of the women having additional or repeat procedures [1, 5].

A multicompartimental (low urinary tract, vagina, and recto-anal compartments) and pluridisciplinary (clinical and functional assessment, imaging, physiotherapy, surgery, etc.) approach to management is usually indicated. Indeed, 95 % of the women involved have complex PFDs involving both the anterior and posterior compartments [5, 6].

The usual assessment of perineal and pelvic floor trauma is clinical, based on a gynaecologic exam. It involves gathering information about symptoms, assessing their impact on quality of life and clinical evaluation of cervico-urethral mobility, prolapse, genital hiatus, perineal body, sphincter, and pelvic floor muscle contraction [7]. Imaging modalities have been used since the middle of last century to assess evidence of types of dysfunction that are not directly accessible by clinical examination such as opening or mobility of the bladder neck [8], impaired elevation of the bladder neck during contraction of the levator [9], weak uterine support by the levator [10], or defects of the anal sphincters [11]. In recent years, ultrasound (US) [12] and magnetic resonance imaging (MRI) [13] have gradually replaced traditional imagery (cystourethrography and colpocystogram) in the study of perineal trauma.

The purpose of this chapter is to describe the modern imaging techniques for the pelvic floor, to clarify expectations and limitations, and to suggest a strategy designed to improve imaging use in everyday practice.

Ultrasound Scan

Technical Ultrasound Aspects

Endocavitary Ultrasound

The endoanal probe is used primarily for study of the anal sphincter and has been the gold standard in case of sphincter lesions. The endoanal ultrasound is performed with a high frequency probe (7.5–10 MHz) to obtain a 360° image of the anal channel, centred on the lumen (Fig. 7.1). Endoanal ultrasound has sensitivity close to 100 % for the diagnosis of anal sphincter injuries (Fig. 7.2). It allows, in 2D or 3D, 360° visualization of the internal anal sphincter (IAS) and of the external anal sphincter (EAS), with good interobserver reliability. However, it is rarely used for study of the pelvic floor.

The transvaginal probe is used to study cervico-urethral mobility [14]. Nevertheless, an intra-vaginal probe situation induces an elevation of the bladder neck at rest and limits its descent during the Valsalva manoeuvre, thereby restricting interpretation of the scan [15]. While the endo-urethral probe helps to distinguish the striated muscle from the smooth muscle in the urethra, it is not used in routine practice [16].

Introital Ultrasound

During an introital ultrasound, the transvaginal probe is placed just below the urethral meatus (to study the urethra), or just above the fourchette (to study the anal sphincter) at the entrance of the vagina [17]. This measurement method was first described as a means of visualising the mobility of the cervico-urethral junction and as a replacement for cystourethrography. Despite the good definition of images, maintaining the stability of the introital probe during cough or Valsalva could be challenging and necessitates a highly skilled operator.

Introital 3D Ultrasound is used to visualize the anal sphincter [18]. The introital position of the probe avoids distortion of the anal canal, including the anal mucosa observed by the endo-rectal probe [19]. Anal sphincter introital ultrasound is performed on a patient in a supine position with a transvaginal probe (or 5-or 6–9 MHz 12 MHz), applied to the vulvar fourchette. 3D acquisitions of the anal sphincter are then performed in the transverse plane allowing a secondary review of the scan on multiplanar cuts.

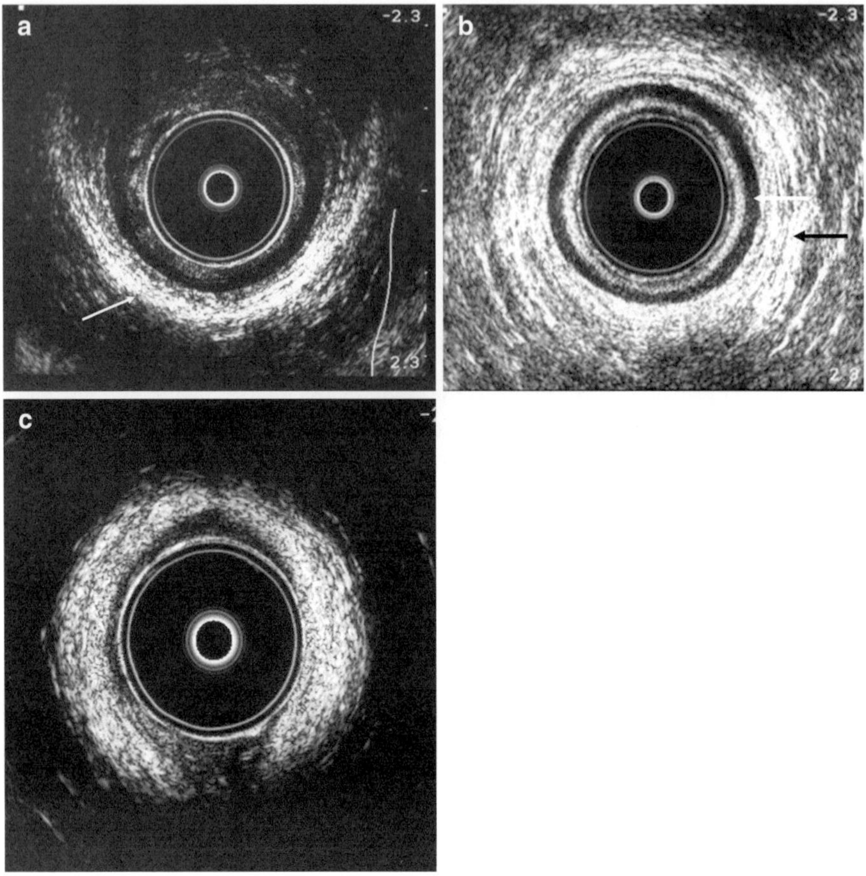

Fig. 7.1 Endoanal scan of the anal sphincter using a 360° rotating 10 MHz probe. (**a**) At the level of the levator: endoanal scan demonstrating the "U"-shaped puborectalis muscle (*white arrow*). (**b**) At the middle of the sphincter: endoanal scan demonstrating the internal anal sphincter (*white arrow*) and the external anal sphincter (*black arrow*). (**c**) Distally: subcutaneous part of the external anal sphincter

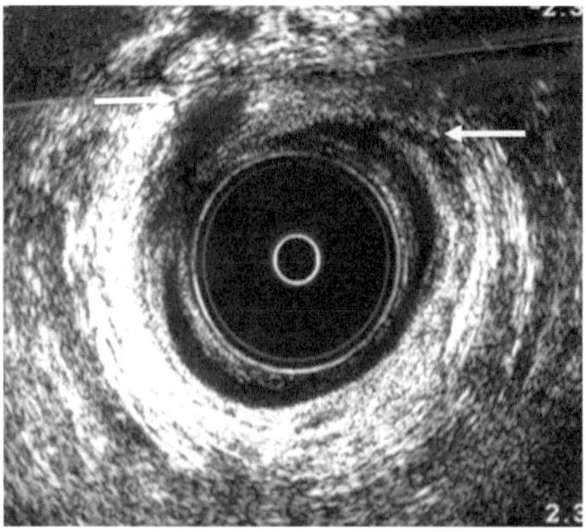

Fig. 7.2 Anal sphincter injury. Endoanal scan with a 360° rotating probe, complete defect of the internal and external anal sphincter from 10 to 2 o'clock (*white arrows*)

Perineal Ultrasound

This is the most widely studied method [20], and the one the authors prefer to assess urethral mobility. During a perineal (or translabial) ultrasound, an abdominal ultrasound probe is placed sagittally on the perineum. This way shows a good correlation with measurements of the urethrovesical angle by cystourethrography, and is less invasive and non-irradiating [21]. It provides a panoramic view of the pelvic organs (Fig. 7.3) and, unlike endocavitary probes, it does not modify the anatomical relationship between the urethra and the surrounding structures [20].

For perineal ultrasound, we use a convex probe of 3.5–5 MHz frequency, protected by a glove applied to the perineum sagittally in contact with the anterior portion of the vestibule without excessive pressure. Ultrasound measurements are performed at rest, during Valsalva manoeuvre, while coughing and during levator contraction [22]. During cough or Valsalva, enough pressure should be applied to maintain a constant scan image while accepting the fact that there is tendency for the probe to be repelled by the prolapse.

Ultrasound scans are usually carried out in a lithotomy or semi-sitting position. Bladder volume should be specified. In our practice, we prefer that the bladder and rectum be largely or totally empty so that the mobility of other organs is not impeded and so that bladder or rectal urgency, which generates artefacts, be limited to the greatest possible extent. For interpretation of the scan, it is essential to observe the pubis, the bladder, the bladder neck and the urethra on a sagittal plane; with a little experience, it is also possible to observe the vagina, the cervix, the rectum and the anal canal (Fig. 7.3). In experienced hands, three-dimensional reconstructions can produce images in the axial plane of the pelvic floor that are almost as accurate as MRI, particularly for evaluation of the urogenital hiatus and the levator muscle (Fig. 7.4) [23, 24].

As is the case with MRI, dynamic study requires perfect cooperation of the patient. It is facilitated by the proximity of the operator with the patient. The use of "frame" function facilitates selection of the snapshot showing the largest

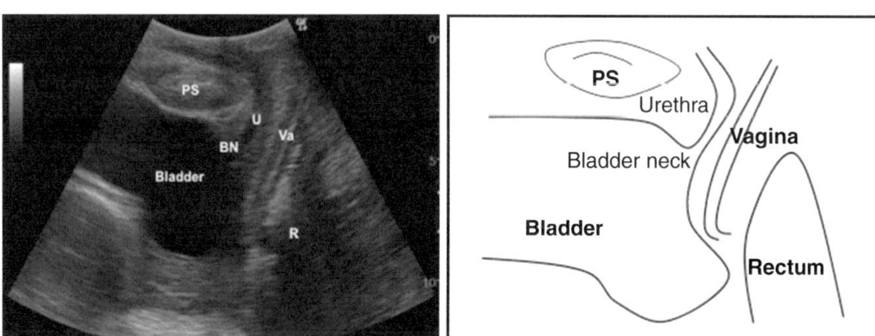

Fig. 7.3 Perineal ultrasound. Sagittal plane with pubis symphysis (*PS*), bladder and bladder neck (*BN*), urethra (*U*), vagina (*Va*), and rectum (*R*) (Extract from: Deffieux X, Fatton B, Amarenco G, de Tayrac R. Manuel pratique d'urogynécologie, pages 37–52. Copyright © 2011 Elsevier Masson SAS. All rights reserved)

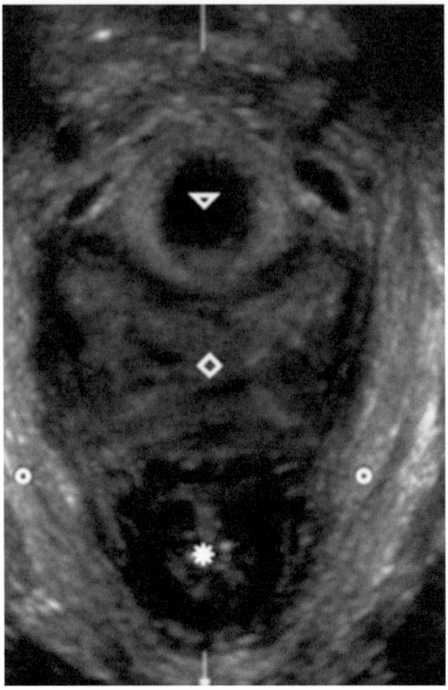

Fig. 7.4 Pelvic floor 3D ultrasound axial scan including pubis, urethra (▼), vagina (✳), anal canal (◇), and levator ani (O)

displacement. The entire scan takes about 10 min. Static and dynamic images can be recorded and then analysed. Acquisition of a dynamic volume at rest and push takes only a few minutes.

Ultrasound Interpretation

Ultrasound Static Measures

Ultrasound Imaging of the Urethra and Bladder

Schaer et al. [16] used an endourethral probe to correlate ultrasound images with histological findings made on cadavers. They individualized a hypoechoic inner layer (internal longitudinal fibers) and a hyperechoic outer layer (circular associated with striated layers smooth fibers). The mucosa and lamina propria containing (submucosa) venous plexus resultantly appear hyperechoic and are not distinguishable from each other. Using perineal ultrasound, the urethral mucosa and submucosa appear hypoechoic.

Athanasiou et al. made 3D scans using an endovaginal probe [25]. They described the urethral sphincter as a "target" anechoic urethral lumen surrounded by a central zone corresponding to hyperechoic smooth internal sphincter and a hypoechoic ring corresponding to the external sphincter of the urethra. The thickness of the sphincter measured by endourethral probe varies between 2.5 and 3.9 mm for the smooth muscle layer and between 2.6 and 3.4 mm for the striated muscle layer [16, 26]. It is possible to measure the volume of the urethral sphincter using a 3D–probe. Before delivery, the volume of the sphincter is correlated with the area under the urethral profile curve [27].

Ultrasound allows measurement of bladder wall thickness [28]. The measurements have yet to be standardised [29]. Average bladder wall thickness greater than 5 mm is associated with a higher risk of detrusor overactivity [30]. The role of bladder wall thickness measurement in clinical practice is still debated. It seems that in case of overactive bladder, monitoring bladder neck wall thickness do not help predicting response to treatment [31].

Ultrasound is the gold standard for assessing post-void residual or track expansion of the pelvicalyceal system possibly secondary to large cystocele or surgery.

Ultrasound Imaging of the Anal Sphincter

Endoanal ultrasound perfectly reflects the concentric layers in the structure of the anal sphincter as anatomically described: the mucosa appears hyperechoic, the internal sphincter hypoechoic, and the external sphincter hyperechoic (Fig. 7.1).

The anal scan may be performed using an introital probe (see section "Obstetrical Perineal Tears") [32]. The technique has been shown to be reproducible at the level of both morphological and biometrical analysis [18, 33]. Introital (or perineal) ultrasound helps to produce images of the anal sphincter; however, its sensitivity seems slightly lower than endoanal ultrasound in detection of lesions of the anal sphincter. Cornelia et al. compared perineal ultrasound to endoanal ultrasound. They found a sensitivity of 50 % for perineal ultrasound. [34] More recently, the PREDICT study, comparing 2D introital and endoanal scan, showed sensitivity and specificity for the diagnosis of anal sphincter lesion of 64 % and 85 %, respectively [35]. Furthermore, using 3D introital scan, sensitivity and specificity are likely to increase, but more clinical studies are still needed [36].

The ultrasound signs on introital scan that were associated with anal sphincter lesion are: interruption of EAS and/or IAS, thickness modification (with a thinner part at the level of the interruption and a thicker part on the opposite side, which has been described as the "half-moon sign"), a loss of the star aspect of the anal canal mucosa [37, 38]. Interobserver reliability for the diagnosis of anal sphincter lesion was good, ranging between 0.80 and 0.95 [39].

Ultrasound Imaging of the Levator Ani

Using a 3D perineal probe, it is also possible to measure the levator hiatus and to identify tears or avulsion of the levator ani (Fig. 7.5). At rest, the levator hiatus has a mean area of 11.4 cm^2 (range 6–36) on nullipara and 14.6 cm^2 on multipara women (see section "Levator Ani Function") [40, 41].

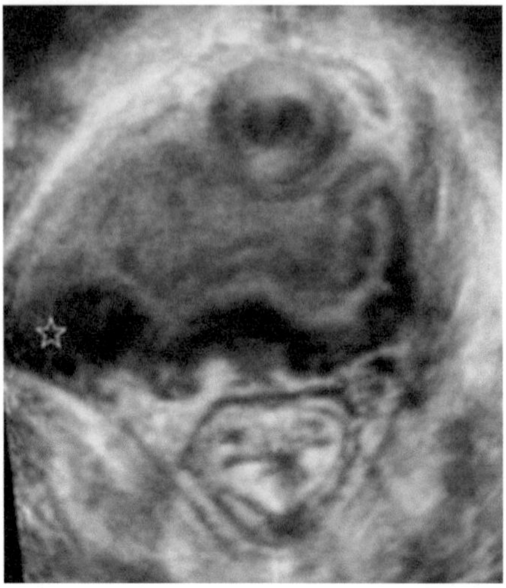

Fig. 7.5 Pelvic floor ultrasound 3D scan, avulsion of the levator ani on one side (★)

Van Delft et al. have studied the inter and intra-observer reproducibility of measurements of the hiatus surface and of levator ani muscle thickness, during pregnancy, just after delivery, and 3 months postpartum in primiparous patients. They reported very good inter and intra observer reproducibility for the measurement of the hiatus surface [42].

Ultrasound Dynamic Measures

Urethra and Bladder Neck Mobility Using Ultrasound

With perineal ultrasound it is easy to measure the position of the bladder neck at rest and during stress, and to assess bladder neck mobility. A number of sonographic parameters have been described, including the posterior urethrovesical angle (UVP) and mobility of the bladder neck on two axes (pubic axis and perpendicular) [43]. The inferior-posterior edge of the symphysis pubis is very easy to distinguish in all women and is used as a fixed anatomical landmark in case of dynamic measurements (Fig. 7.6) [21]. In our practice, this benchmark is of proven reliability in verification of the absence of involuntary mobilization of the probe during dynamic movements.

Using perineal ultrasound, Dietz proposed to simplify the measurement of the mobility of the bladder neck by measuring the Bladder Neck Descent (BND) on the axis of the perineal probe during Valsalva manoeuvre. He measured bladder neck displacement along the probe axis and neglected lateral bladder neck displacement (Fig. 7.7). BND distance corresponds to the subtraction of distances BSD (bladder symphyseal distance or distance between the symphysis pubis and the bladder neck) at rest and Valsalva manoeuvre. He found excellent reproducibility of the measurement [44]. In our clinical practice, the latter is relatively easy to achieve and appears somewhat correlated with clinical measurement of the mobility of point Aa (In the POP-Q system, point Aa is located at rest 3 cm inside the vagina, just under

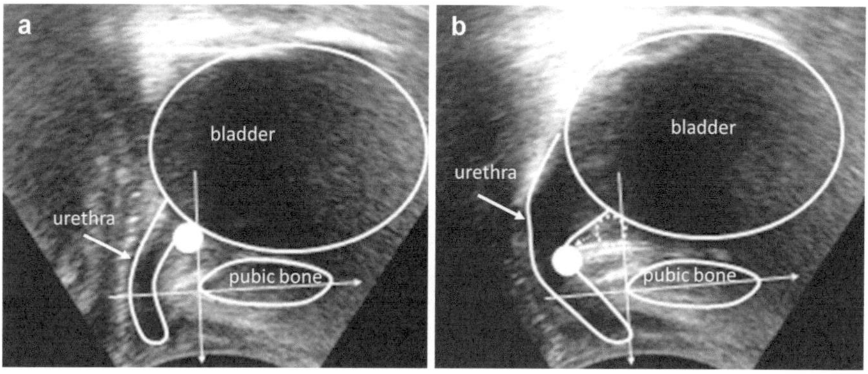

Fig. 7.6 Ultrasound scan, bladder neck mobility. Perineal ultrasound for evaluation of bladder neck mobility. Bladder neck at rest (**a**) and with Valsalva (**b**), point indicates the bladder neck, arrow as vector for bladder neck mobility

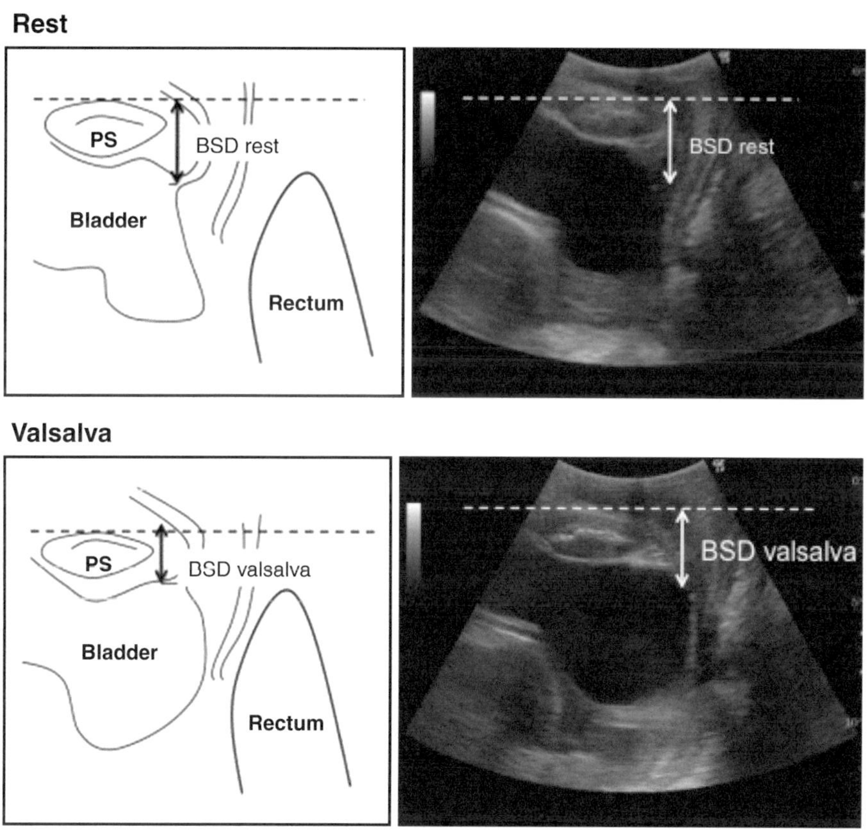

Fig. 7.7 Ultrasound scan, bladder neck descent (Dietz measure). Bladder-Symphyseal Distance (*BSD*): the distance of the bladder neck relative to the horizontal line through the lower edge of the pubic symphysis (*PS*), at rest and during Valsalva (mm). Bladder Neck Descent (*BND*): difference between rest and strain (*BSD rest – BSD Valsalva,* mm) (Extract from: Deffieux X, Fatton B, Amarenco G, de Tayrac R. Manuel pratique d'urogynécologie, pages 37–52.)

the bladder neck. The measurement of clinical urethral mobility, recorded during maximum strain with respect to the hymen, is negative if located within the hymen and positive if located outside. It varies between −3 and +3 cm). Unfortunately, detailed information on inter or intra observer reproducibility is currently lacking. Our opinion is that reproducibility of the measurement might be impaired by two factors. First it is difficult to maintain the placement of the probe during the Valsalva manoeuvre. Second it may be difficult draw a definite line to measure BND. Proper evaluation will be needed in future studies.

There is no unanimously accepted definition of normal values for cervico-urethral mobility. However, it appears acceptable to use a BND threshold value of 15–20 mm to define cervico-urethral hypermobility [44–46].

Pelvic Organ Mobility Using Ultrasound

The mobility of the bladder, uterus, rectum and pouch of Douglas may be measured according to the same principle as when measuring the descent of the bladder neck [20, 47, 48]. Dietz et al. compared the clinical examination based on POP-Q classification and perineal ultrasound in 145 symptomatic patients. They found a good statistical correlation for uterine prolapse and anterior vaginal prolapse. The correlation between ultrasound and clinical examination, however, appears moderate for posterior vaginal prolapse [49]. Similar results have been found by Broekhuis et al. using 3D ultrasound [50]. The main problem with ultrasound in this context is incomplete visualization of the cervix and uterus when there is a large rectocele and possible underestimation of large prolapse related to the probe pressure on the perineum [20].

Kluivers et al. compared ultrasound to clinical examination (POP-Q) and found that clinical examination better predicted symptoms of prolapse than ultrasound. However, ultrasound allowed the authors to distinguish between enteroceles or rectoceles and rectal intussusception [51]. In fact, perineal ultrasound renders it possible to visualize the intrarectal prolapse.

Levator Ani Function Using Ultrasound

One advantage of ultrasound resides in visualisation of the levator ani muscle during voluntary contraction or Valsalva manoeuvre. A reflex contraction of the levator may occur during the Valsalva manoeuvre, and because this reflex contraction may decrease the mobility of the bladder neck, it needs to be taken into account when interpreting measurements of bladder neck mobility [52].

The levator hiatus can be studied during effort or contraction. Dietz et al. reviewed datasets of 544 women seen in an urogynecological unit for pelvic floor or lower urinary tract symptoms. They considered abnormal a hiatus of more than 25 cm^2 during the Valsalva manoeuvre [53].

Variation of the levator hiatus (or reduction of the anteroposterior diameter) between rest and voluntary contraction is sometimes used to quantify contraction of the pelvic floor [54]. Dietz et al. estimated contraction of the levator muscles by measuring the displacement of the urethral meatus. It seems that the use of perineal ultrasound biofeedback facilitates understanding by patients of the effect of perineal muscle contraction and thereby renders their training more effective [55].

Magnetic Resonance Imaging (MRI)

Technical MRI Aspects

Subject Position During MRI

Dynamic MRI is classically carried out with patients in supine position and flexed legs [12, 56]. Dynamic MRIs with opened antennas are now available to achieve the acquisitions in a standing or a sitting position with defecation [57]. It is not certain that imaging in a standing position improves its relevance. The only study comparing sitting position in an open-magnet unit versus supine position in a closed-magnet unit did not conclude that the sitting position presented a clear advantage [58].

Organ Opacification, Bladder Filling and MRI

Due to spontaneous high resolution (hyper signal T2) and high contrasts on MRI (Fig. 7.8), the bladder and the vagina do not need opacification [59, 60–62]. The bladder has to be semi-filled to be easily identified; if it is overfilled, anatomical relationships can be modified and the diagnosis may change due to competition for space between pelvic organs [63]. In practice we recommend emptying of the bladder half an hour before the examination. Usually, the vaginal walls are easily recognized by MRI without need for vaginal highlighting; use of 10–50 ml of sterile ultrasound gel modifies fewer anatomical relationships than a tampon, which does not usually remain medial.

The need for opacification of the rectum is debated. Some teams prefer to fill the rectum with mashed potatoes or gadolinium-DPTA [64]. For them, this method avoids collapse of the anterior wall and enhances rectocele diagnosis. However, filling may increase competition for space and leads to underdiagnosis of compressed pelvic organ prolapse. Excessive rectal filling can also modify the anatomy of the pelvic organs [63]. Rectal gel can also aggravate a feeling of discomfort characterized by fear of the occurrence of faecal leak during the effort. For our point of view, it is rather easy to precisely quantify rectocele without rectal opacification because of rectal gas, which appear in black [65]. Lakeman et al. in a cross-sectional study of symptomatic women with and without prolapse, showed good reproducibility for the posterior compartment measurement in the prolapse group without rectal opacification [62].

Static sequences are obtained using T2-weighted axial and sagittal planes that give a precise three-plane morphologic analysis while dynamic sequences are produced using single-slice ultrafast acquisitions in sagittal and coronal planes. The T2-weighted sagittal sequences help to highlight the bladder neck and the cervix

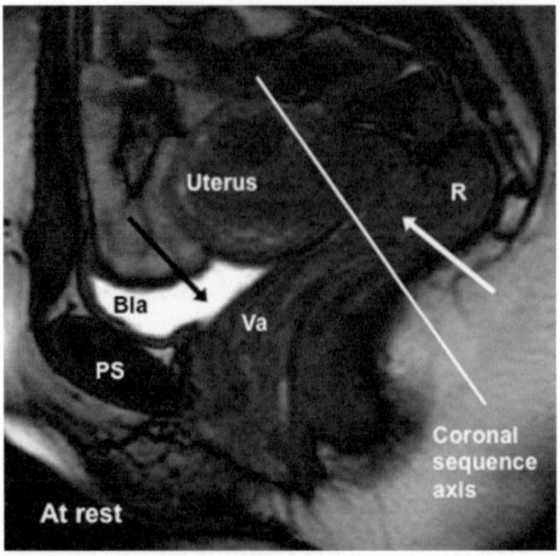

Fig. 7.8 MRI visualisation of the bladder and the vagina, sagittal plane. MRI T2-weighted sagittal sequences with pubic symphysis (*PS*), bladder neck (*black arrow*) and uterine cervix (*white arrow*). On MRI T2-weighted sequences, the bladder (*Bla*) and the vagina (*Va*) appear with high resolution without any opacification. Stepped appearance of pelvic viscera: the uterine body depends on the bladder, bladder into the vagina, the vagina and cervix to the rectum (*R*) and the anal canal (Extract from: Deffieux X, Fatton B, Amarenco G, de Tayrac R. Manuel pratique d'urogynécologie, pages 37–52. Copyright © 2011 Elsevier Masson SAS. All rights reserved)

(Fig. 7.8). Sagittal acquisitions help to adjust coronal images while identifying the middle passing through the pubic symphysis and the anatomical landmarks. They also facilitate precise morphologic analysis. Coronal planes explore dynamic contraction of the elevator muscles (Fig. 7.9) [66].

Dynamic sequences are obtained on a sagittal plane in different positions: restraining, neutral pushing and at times defecation (see section "Defecation"). Some authors have compiled sequences after defecation in toilets [67].

Valsalva Manoeuvres During MRI

Valsalva manoeuvres need to be standardized, explained to the patients and repeated to obtain a maximal prolapse [68]. Standard manoeuvres consist of several repeated cycles of maximal and sustained straining. The cycles are monitored and repeated until the same degree of protrusion observed during the MRI sequence remains constant at least three times [59]. Patients are also instructed in the Valsalva manoeuvre before the beginning of the examination and instructions are repeated for each imaging sequence [59, 69].

Speculum Use During MRI

Some authors suggest using speculum valves during dynamic MRI to expose compartments at risk of prolapse during strain or Valsalva manoeuvres and to increase the rate of detection of posterior compartment prolapse in patients

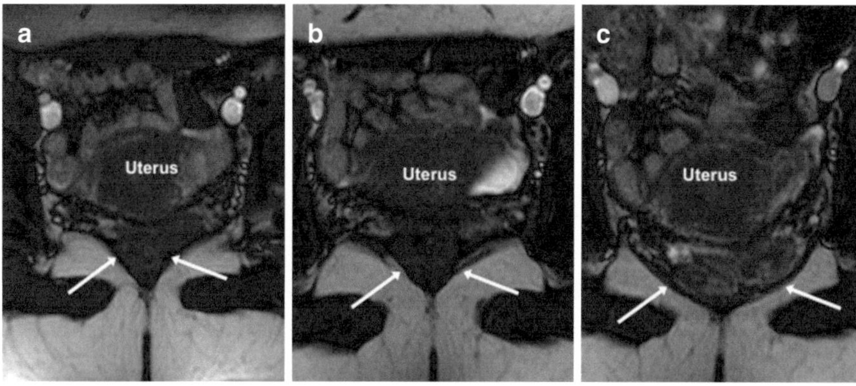

Fig. 7.9 Dynamic MRI coronal planes of the levator ani muscles (*white arrows*). At rest, the levator ani muscles have the aspect of a convex dome. (**b**) During levator ani contraction (restrain), there is a horizontalisation of muscle fascicles. (**c**) During Valsalva manoeuvre, bloated muscles allowing for expansion of the pelvic hiatus (Extract from: Deffieux X, Fatton B, Amarenco G, de Tayrac R. Manuel pratique d'urogynécologie, pages 37–52. Copyright © 2011 Elsevier Masson SAS. All rights reserved)

with voluminous cystoceles [70]. Indeed, during physical examination a speculum is routinely used to assess each vaginal compartment separately in order to detect occult POP components [71]. Using a speculum during examination is likely to change the nature of the prolapse. Competition for space between the different components of POP may produce compartment overlapping; for example a cystocele will hold the posterior wall in place. Use of a speculum is never performed during routine MRI examination for obvious reasons such as discomfort, and extended examination time. This restriction may explain the discrepancies between MRI examination and clinical examination of women with POP [59, 67].

Defecation During MRI

Some teams consider MR defecography sequences as a part of dynamic MRI arguing that adequate straining and defecation guarantee better visualization of prolapse and anorectal disease [72]. Dynamic MR defecography sequences may indeed be helpful in case of defecation disorders. It requires opacification of the rectum, before or during the examination. Defecation is considered adequate if rectal material is evacuated with a changing anorectal angle. Nevertheless, in a study of ten women, no correlation was found between MRI defecography and conventional defecography in anorectal angle at rest or straining [73]. Comparing sequences before and after rectopexy on 21 patients, Otto et al. found that changes in the anorectal angle are less sizable in MRI defecography than with conventional defecography during squeezing and evacuation [74]. These differences may arise from the supine position used in MR defecography resulting contrary to cinedefecography in a lack of gravity.

For rectal intussusceptions, evacuation proctography appears preferable to dynamic defecography. A comparative study on ten patients showed underestimation by MRI of intussusception and rectocele size. However, MRI more clearly differentiates full thickness than mucosal intussusception and provides overall information on the pelvis [75]. Foti et al. compared evacuation proctography to MRI defecography with or without evacuation. Adjunction of an evacuation phase in MRI facilitates detection of rectocele, perineal descent as effectively as evacuation proctography [76].

MRI Interpretation

Regular MRI Results

At rest, using T2 sequences, in sagittal plane, the bladder has a homogeneous fluid content that appears hyperintense; its walls are hypointense and of uniform thickness. The bladder neck is usually visible on top of the pubococcygeal line on account of its V-shaped appearance (Fig. 7.8). The urethra appears attached to the anterior wall of the vagina. Its middle part is vertical, joining the bladder neck forming the urethrovesical angle. On the other hand, the vaginal walls appear hypointense with vesicovaginal and rectovaginal spaces at times underlined by a greasy hyperintense border (T2). The appearance of the rectum depends on its content; for example, gas appears black when visualizing the rectal wall (Fig. 7.8). When using ultrasound gel intrarectally, however, it appears hyperintense (T2). The anal canal is made up of different layers: mucosa hyperintense, submucosa hypointense, internal sphincter hyperintense on T2, and external sphincter hypointense. The pouch of Douglas, located between the uterus and the rectum, visibility depends on its fat content.

Using axial T2 sequences, the anatomy of the urethra is particularly well-displayed with a central hyperintense area corresponding to the mucosa, a low signal corresponding to the submucosa, the hyperintense smooth muscle, and peripherally the hypointense striated muscle [77]. The pubo-visceral portion (or pubo-rectalis) of the levator ani muscle is recognized using axial T2 sequences by its U-shape. It forms a belt around the pelvic organs and joins its contralateral fellow behind the anorectal junction (Fig. 7.10). Measurements of the urogenital hiatus can be performed on axial planes: the transverse diameter corresponds to the inter-pubo-rectalis distance and the anteroposterior diameter of the urogenital hiatus is the lower edge of the pubis at the posterior part of the anal canal. However, these measurements have large inter-individual variability. A study of 23 young nulliparous women found asymptomatic measurements between 26 and 46 mm for the internal transverse diameter and between 29 and 48 mm for the anteroposterior diameter [78].

During Valsalva manoeuvre, using sagittal T2, the bladder undergoes a movement down and back; the bladder neck also translates down and the mid-urethra horizontalizes; the posterior urethrovesical angle opens and almost completely disappears. While the urethral meatus is a fixed point in the lower edge of the

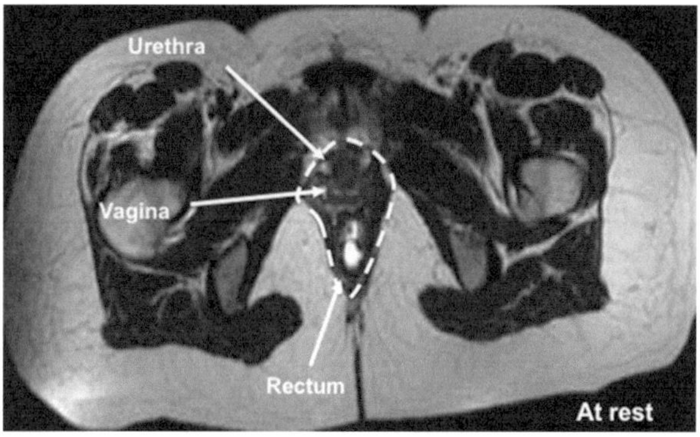

Fig. 7.10 MRI T2, axial plane, the levator hiatus (*dotted line*) (Extract from: Deffieux X, Fatton B, Amarenco G, de Tayrac R. Manuel pratique d'urogynécologie, pages 37–52. Copyright © 2011 Elsevier Masson SAS. All rights reserved)

pubis [79], the uterus becomes vertical and cervix moves down and back. The vagina becomes straight, leading to the disappearance of its cap. The rectum falls, becomes vertical and tends to align with the anal canal. All three pelvic viscera, bladder, cervical and vaginal dome and the rectum are projected rearward against the bottom and the median raphe, which becomes vertical. Using coronal T2, all three pelvic viscera press upon the pelvic floor. The iliococcygeal parts of the levator ani muscle flatten to become concave with maximal upward thrust [80].

During levator contraction, on a sagittal plane, the levator ani muscles bring the median pelvic organs upward and forward; the posterior urethrovesical angle and the vaginal cap close, while the rectum and the median raphe become horizontal; on the coronal plane, the convexity of the levator ani muscles disappears, reflecting isometric muscle contraction (Fig. 7.9) [80]. On the axial plane, the diameter of the urogenital hiatus is decreased by bringing together the pubo-rectal portions of the levator ani muscles. [80].

Quantitative Measures of Mobility and Pelvic Organ Prolapse Using MRI

Several lines are used to provide MRI POP classification (Table 7.1, Fig. 7.11) [12, 58, 81–83]. Lakeman et al. assessed the interobserver agreement of four different lines: the pubococcygeal line (PCL), the midpubic line (MPL), the perineal line (PL), and the H-line in three groups of ten women (two groups of symptomatic women with or without prolapse and nulliparous women). They showed good to excellent agreement for anterior and middle compartment in the three groups of women for the PCL, MPL and H-Line. For the posterior compartment, agreement for the four lines was good only in the prolapse group [62]. Reproducibility depends not only on the pelvic compartment but also on patients. We have compared the PL to the MPL (inter-and intra-observer variability) and it was found that in practice the midpubic line was easier to draw than the perineal line [59]. In general the positions of the different points measuring POP quantification by MRI dynamic image were very easy to place and have good reproducibility [59].

Table 7.1 Lines used for MRI interpretation

Reference line	Definition	Advantages/drawbacks
Pubococcygeal line (PCL)	Yang (1991) [13]	Reproducible and independent of pelvis tilting
	Most useful reference line in pelvic floor disorders	Good correlation between PCL and classification of prolapse for anterior and middle compartments
	Inferioposterior margin of the pubic symphysis to the anterior margin Corresponds to levator plate	But Lieneman et al. [61] found a correlation only for anterior compartment
Midpubic line (MPL)	Singh (2001) [81]	A major drawback is that the quantification of the prolapse depends on the difference of points through this line at straining and at rest
	Also called hymeneal line	Two measurements for one point are necessary increasing the risk of intra and inter observatory differences
	Line drawn through the longitudinal axis of the pubic bone and passing through its midequatorial point	Correlation between prolapse grades and imaging is only moderate
	On cadaveric dissections, it corresponds to the hymen	This line may be used only for the posterior compartment Hymen is mobile
Perineal line (PL)	Fauconnier (2008) [59] Line as tangent from the internal surface from the symphysis pubis down to the caudal end of the internal sphincter	Correlation with clinical exam is not major
Line passing through the anterior margin of the anal canal	Yoshioka (1991) [82] Enables assessment of prolapse from digestive compartment Follows axis of the anterior margin of anal canal	Under variation because anal canal is sometimes difficult to visualize without defecation
H-line	Comiter (1999) [83] Horizontal tangent of the inferior rim of the pubic bone. It corresponds to a sagittal plane passing through the midline at the level of the ischiatic tubera, which is the reference in prolapse in colpocystodefecography	It can change in case of straining or tilting

Levator Ani Assessment Using MRI

MRI authorizes diagnosis of levator ani defects or avulsions and measurement of the levator hiatus. Lammers et al. found good interobserver reliability for the diagnosis of avulsions and excellent agreement for measurements of the levator hiatus.

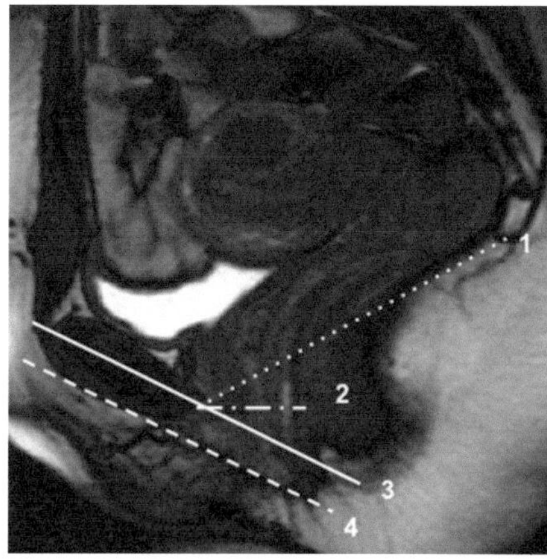

Fig. 7.11 MRI prolapse staging, Different reference line used. (*1*) Pubococcygeal line [13]. (*2*) H-Line [83]. (*3*) Midpubic line [81]. (*4*) Perineal line [59] (Extract from: Deffieux X, Fatton B, Amarenco G, de Tayrac R. Manuel pratique d'urogynécologie, pages 37–52. Copyright © 2011 Elsevier Masson SAS. All rights reserved)

Intraobserver reliability for avulsions and levator hiatus measurements was also excellent [84].

Role of Imaging in Clinical Practice

Urethral Function

Perineal ultrasound can easily explore cervico-urethral mobility [20]. Dynamic MRI, as well as ultrasound, allow the study of urethral mobility, bladder neck opening at stress, and cervico-urethral angle on the condition that the examination be performed correctly. Published studies validating this indication for MRI are nonetheless lacking, so it is not indicated for urinary symptoms alone.

The measurement of bladder neck descent (proposed by Dietz) appears to be the ultrasound parameter most significantly associated with urinary incontinence [85]. Similarly, in a case-control study Pregazzi et al. measured the urethral mobility in relation to the distance between the bladder neck and the inferior-posterior symphysis in 23 incontinent women and 50 controls. They found higher urethral mobility during Valsalva manoeuvre and cough among incontinent women [86]. However, not all authors have found this difference significant [46]. There is also an overlap in measurements of urethral mobility in incontinent and continent women. Dietz found values ranging between 1 and 40 mm for the measurement BND in 106 nulliparous continent women [47]. Ultrasound measurement of cervico-urethral mobility is of highly variable prognostic validity in assessing the severity of SUI. Bai et al. did not reveal any significant difference between ultrasound parameters according to the severity of SUI [46]. Their findings do not justify diagnosis of stress urinary incontinence by simple measurement of cervico-urethral mobility.

In patients with stress urinary incontinence, a wide neck opening can be seen on ultrasound during the Valsalva manoeuvre (funnelling). Some studies have found an association between funnelling of the cervix and low urethral closure pressure [87, 88]. However, the opening of the cervix is not specific and can also be found in continent women, particularly multiparous women [89]. It therefore cannot characterize stress urinary incontinence.

Kim et al. used an endocavitary MRI antenna to measure the urethral striated muscle and the pubo-rectal muscles among continent and incontinent women. They found a significant difference in the thickness of the striated muscle between the two groups as well as frequent asymmetries of the pubo-rectal muscles in incontinent patients [90]. However, Tunn et al. showed that the pelvic floor muscle changes found on MRI in patients with incontinence are not correlated with clinical parameters. For these authors, they have no direct link with urinary incontinence [91].

Overall, the only indication of urethral mobility assessment, using either ultrasound or dynamic MRI, is to search for fixity of the urethra in women requiring secondary surgical procedures, as it is a prognosis factor before sub-urethral sling [92].

Pelvic Organ Prolapse Assessment

The concordance of POP measurements carried out with imaging (ultrasound or MRI) with those performed using clinical examination seems rather poor [51, 59, 61, 62, 93–96].

Imaging Versus Physical Examination for Pelvic Organ Prolapse Assessment

In a prospective study on 30 women with prolapse stage ≥1 according to Baden-Walker classification, Novellas et al. compared clinical examination to the pubococcygeal (PCL) and midpubic lines (MPL). They found a mild to moderate concordance between clinical evaluation and both MRI lines [95]. Lienemann et al. retrospectively compared functional cine-MRI of 41 asymptomatic volunteers with clinical examination using POP-Q. They found a correlation between clinical examination and RMI for anterior compartment using the PCL and posterior compartment using the MPL. They concluded that organ descent on functional cine-MRI cannot be described using only a single reference line [61]. Considering intraoperative findings as the gold standard on 100 consecutive women with and without prolapse, Gousse et al. found high sensitivity, specificity, positive predictive value and negative predictive value for the anterior and middle compartments only [65]. Studying the role of dynamic MRI in the evaluation of vaginal vault prolapse, Cortes et al. found poor correlation between clinical and MRI findings [93]. More recently, Broekhuis et al. prospectively compared the POP-Q points and measurements on dynamic MRI using three different lines (PCL, MPL and H-Line) on 98 women.

The correlations were good to moderate in the anterior compartment and moderate to poor in the central and posterior compartment. This finding was independent of the staging method and reference lines used [94]. Lakeman et al. found good correlation in symptomatic women with prolapse for all the compartments with at least one reference line but a poor correlation in symptomatic women without prolapse. They concluded that prolapse in dynamic MR should be described with several lines and that the added clinical value of such staging is questionable due to poor association with clinical findings and pelvic floor symptoms [62]. In addition, we showed that major individual variability exists between clinical and MRI measures on the same patient with gaps of up to 5 cm whatever line was used [59]. This raises a question about the clinical significance of the observations carried out using MRI. Nevertheless, MRI provides information associated with elongation of the uterine cervix. This scan easily distinguishes two types of cervix elongation: intravaginal elongation and intraperitoneal elongation. To diagnose rectoceles, MRI is more sensitive than clinical examination. In fact, MRI sensitivity varies between 82 % and 100 % vs. 31–80 % for clinical examination [5, 75].

Imaging Versus Prolapse Symptoms

Broekhuis et al. found that the correlation between symptoms and dynamic MRI was poor: the only symptom correlated with the degree of pelvic organ prolapse measured by MRI was the sensation or visualization of a bulge in the vagina [97]. In a critical effort to clarify the relationship between symptoms and clinical or MRI observation, Lakeman et al. designed a very interesting study comparing pelvic floor symptoms assessed by questionnaires to the clinical or MRI observations carried out in two groups with or without POP. They observed a significant but disappointing correlation between urinary incontinence symptoms and prolapse of the middle compartment in their control group without POP. In the POP group, a significant correlation between pain symptoms and prolapse of the posterior compartment assessed using dynamic MRI [62]. While these results are cumulatively weak, an important finding of the study was that the additional diagnostic value of dynamic MRI for staging POP, even in women with unexplained symptoms, seems limited.

MRI Versus Ultrasound for Prolapse Assessment

Few authors have evaluated the correlation between ultrasound and MRI for the staging of prolapse. Broekhuis et al. compared 3D dynamic MRI and ultrasound to POP-Q measurements. They used as a baseline an ultrasound horizontal line passing through the inferior-posterior to the pubic symphysis as described by Dietz [20], and three MRI baselines described above board: the PBL, the H-line and the MPL (Table 7.1). They found good to moderate correlation for the anterior compartment, and poor to moderate correlation for the posterior compartment [50].

3D ultrasound provides easier access at a lower cost than MRI, which might have an added value in research considering its capacity to evaluate the entire pelvis including support structures and organs.

Levator Ani Function

Levator Ani Defects After Vaginal Delivery

Imaging (MRI or ultrasound) can easily visualize pelvic muscle injuries, especially after vaginal birth (Fig. 7.5). Kearney et al. found that 11 % of women who delivered normally and 25–66 % of women who had forceps delivery had evidence of levator ani (LA) injury on MRI [98]. These lesions usually consist of a muscle defect and are most clearly recognized on axial sequences (Fig. 7.11). Using 3D perineal ultrasound, avulsion of the levator ani muscles was significantly associated with measurements of a larger urogenital hiatus, at rest, push and levator contraction [99].

Levator Ani Defects and Prolapse

In the absence of large longitudinal studies, the repercussions of these muscle defects on the prognosis of patients are not clear, but most authors found a correlation with pelvic organ prolapse and levator ani muscle defects [100]. In a case control study, DeLancey et al. found that women with prolapse were more likely to have major levator ani defects compared to women with normal support. They noted LA defects in 77 % of women with anterior compartment prolapse, in 80 % of women with middle compartment prolapse and 48 % of women with posterior compartment prolapse [101]. In a 3D simulation of cystocele formation, the same author found larger cystocele when levator ani and connective tissue impairment were present [102]. In a prospective study using perineal ultrasound on 333 middle-aged women Dietz et al. confirmed, that prolapse of the anterior and middle compartment was more frequent and at higher grades in women with LA avulsion. No association between avulsion and posterior compartment prolapse was found in this study [103]. Other authors studying women with anal sphincter tears noted symptomatic prolapse in 35 % of women with LA avulsion against 15.5 % for women without muscle injury at 12 months after delivery [104].

Levator Ani Defects and Anal Incontinence

It seems that there are more levator ani avulsions in cases of anal incontinence. A study by DeLancey et al. found that women with pubovisceral injuries had more anal sphincter ruptures, but it is not specified whether they had symptoms of anal incontinence [98]. For women with sphincter rupture and avulsion Heilbrun found a higher rate of faecal incontinence (35.5 % vs. 16.7 % in cases of sphincter rupture without avulsion) [104].

Levator Ani Defects and Urinary Incontinence

It seems that LA defects are not associated with stress urinary incontinence [100]. Morgan et al. conducted a prospective study on urinary symptoms in 151 women with prolapse. They were divided into three groups based on MRI findings: levator ani integrity, major and minor trauma. Women with major trauma experienced four times less urinary incontinence than with normal muscle. They explained the difference between minor and major LA trauma with the potentially different associated damages of the pudendal nerve in case of minor or major LA trauma [105].

Obstructive voiding was not associated with the presence of muscle damage [105]. Twelve months after delivery, Heilbrun et al. did not find an association between levator ani trauma (major or minor) and SUI symptoms in 206 primiparous women [104]. In a study on 160 primiparous women 9–12 months after delivery Brincat et al. reported that LA damage was unrelated to urethral pressure profile. They concluded that LA damage during delivery seems to spare the urethra [106].

Perineal ultrasound can also be used to assess the effect of pelvic floor muscle training (PFMT) on pelvic floor. Bernstein et al. measured the thickness of the levator muscles before and after PFMT in incontinent patients. They found a hypertrophy of these muscles after training [107].

Anal Sphincter Function

Ultrasound of the anal sphincter is recommended in patients with anal incontinence when trauma is suspected and if surgery to repair the sphincter is being considered [108]. It helps to objectify sphincter lesions, to locate and assess their extent and type with sensitivity and specificity approaching 100 % [109, 110]. Damage to the internal sphincter appears as a hyperechoic gap in the hypoechoic ring of the muscle. Damage to the external sphincter is defined as a hypoechoic gap in the hyperechoic muscular ring (Fig. 7.2). Starck et al. developed a score to classify the severity of sphincter lesions [111]. Using 2D ultrasound, they found in patients who had undergone immediate repair of tears of the third and fourth degree a positive correlation between the degree of incontinence and the extent of sphincter injury [112].

However, the presence of sphincter lesions visible to the endoanal ultrasound is not synonymous with functional signs of anal incontinence. In a study of 20 nulliparous patients comparing their endoanal ultrasound and anorectal manometry findings Sentovich et al. showed that there could be false positives [113]. They explained this by the fact that in the upper part of the anal canal, the sphincter is anteriorly physiologically incomplete. Three-dimensional ultrasound could rectify this deficiency by allowing reconstruction in three planes of space [114]. That is why this type of scan requires trained operators.

Some studies have compared endoanal ultrasound and MRI in 2D and did not find any significant difference in the diagnosis of sphincter tears [115, 116]. However, MRI is reported as superior to endoanal ultrasound for the diagnosis of sphincter atrophy, an important predictor of sphincteroplasty [115, 117]. The use of 3D ultrasound can overcome this difference since it has the same sensitivity and specificity as MRI in detection of sphincter atrophy [118]. MRI and 3D ultrasound are used to explore the lesions and atrophy of the anal sphincter while giving an overview of the pelvic floor.

Obstetrical Perineal Tears

Introital scan should be useful in the delivery room, just after vaginal delivery, to improve the anal sphincter lesion diagnostic rate. Clinical evaluation was shown to have a relatively poor sensitivity, with poor inter-observer reliability [37]. Six weeks after delivery, the rate of occult anal sphincter lesion shown by endoanal scan was 29–35 % [19]. Improvement of the diagnosis rate is likely to increase the number of anal sphincter sutures, which could decrease the rate of post-partum anal incontinence [119]. These preliminary results have still got to be confirmed by further studies.

Introital scan is well-accepted by patients, in comparison to endoanal scan, and is more accessible to obstetricians (same probe as endovaginal scan) [120].

While there is still no study available with regard to the time of delivery, a few authors have described the use of introital scan close to delivery. Using introital scan 24–72 h after delivery on 139 primiparous women with stage 2 or less perineal tear, Valsky et al. showed analyzable volumes in 91.4 % and entire anal sphincter visualization in 84.6 % of the cases. Among these patients, 7.9 % had occult anal sphincter tears [37]. In another study, on primiparous women with immediate (6–24 h) post-partum anal incontinence, 2D introital scan has shown anal sphincter tear in 89 %. Lesions were partial EAS defect in 93 % and total EAS defect in 7 % [121]. In the latter study, sensitivity and specificity of 2D introital scan for the diagnosis of anal sphincter lesion were 100 % and 94 %, respectively, with positive and negative predictive values of 77 % and 100 %, respectively [121].

Defecation

In case of anorectal dysfunction, MR defecography can reveal various pelvic floor abnormalities, including rectal descent, enterocele, anterior proctocele, and internal rectal prolapse. Hetzer et al. performed open MR defecography in 50 patients with faecal incontinence: it revealed rectal descent of more than 6 cm (relative to the pubococcygeal line) in all women. Vaginal vault descent of more than 3 cm was present in 19 (43 %) of 44 women. Moreover, 17 (34 %) anterior proctoceles, 16 (32 %) enteroceles and 10 (20 %) rectal prolapses were noted. Interobserver agreement was good to excellent (0.6–0.91) for image analysis results. MR defecography findings led to changes in the surgical approach in 22 (67 %) of 33 patients who had undergone surgery [122].

Surgical Results

Ultrasound has been used to study the results of Burch colposuspension. Viereck et al. found a significant decrease in cervical mobility using introital ultrasound after colposuspension in 310 women. Postoperative hypermobility was significantly associated with a high recurrence rate of urinary incontinence at 6 months and 4 years after surgery [123]. Martan et al. compared ultrasound parameters in 70 incontinent women and 52 women undergoing retropubic colposuspension. They found a significant difference between the two groups in the distance between the bladder neck and pubic symphysis. In operated women, de novo urge incontinence and postoperative voiding obstruction were significantly correlated with detrusor thickness >5 mm and a low urethral mobility [124].

The risk of failure after mid-urethra tape increases when preoperative urethral mobility is low [92]. Sarlos et al. found a kinking of the urethra at stress and a compression of the tissue between the mid-urethra tape and the symphysis pubis without any change in the urethrovesical junction. Suburethral plication appears to contribute to postoperative continence [125]. Masata et al. found a significant decrease in the cervico-urethral mobility after suburethral sling [126].

In a study of 54 patients with suburethral sling, Ducarme et al. found a correlation between voiding dysfunction observed at 3 months postoperatively (obstructive voiding, urge incontinence) and the distance between the tape and the bladder neck [127].

There is a higher risk of prolapse recurrence after surgery in case of LA defects [128, 129]. Morgan et al. reviewed post-operative outcomes according to levator ani defect status determined by MRI on 107 women: they found that women with major LA avulsions were less likely to have anterior compartment support compared to women with no or minor avulsion [128]. This finding was confirmed in the prospective study by Weemhoff et al. on 122 women 31 months after surgery (with perineal ultrasonography) where 52 % of women with anatomical recurrence of cystocele had complete LA avulsion compared to 31 % of women without anatomical recurrence [130].

Tape and Mesh

MRI is inferior to ultrasound as a means of finding Tension free Vaginal Tape (TVT) around the urethra. MRI nevertheless seems to be superior as a means of visualising the retropubic part of the tape [131]. Using MRI to search tape placed by obturator way is usually not adapted except in the event of infection or inflammatory complications of vaginal tape, in which the vaginal tape is surrounded by a hypersignal T1 after injection of gadolinium and T2 and MRI can diagnose hematoma, abscess and myositis.

Concerning prolapse surgery, vaginal and rectal meshes positioned vaginally or laparoscopically are well-visualised by MRI or ultrasound. Imaging is interesting in case of recurrence after primary surgery with meshes. It visualises the spreading, coverage of meshes and moving of pelvic organs. The anatomical corrections have been well-studied.

Ultrasound may be useful to assess the postoperative retraction of meshes. Using introital ultrasound Tunn et al. found a decrease of up to 50 % in the length of the mesh 6 weeks after cystocele or rectocele vaginal repair [132]. Letouzey et al. studied long-term sub-bladder polypropylene meshes using 3D perineal ultrasound. They found 30 % shrinkage at three postoperative years, 65 % within 6 years. For over 8 years, some prostheses represent only 15 % of the initial surface [133].

Conclusion

Imaging scans such as MRI or perineal ultrasound effectively contribute to morphological and functional analysis of the pelvic floor.

Dynamic MRI provides an overall qualitative assessment of the pelvic floor and pelvic organ prolapse. It achieves excellent differentiation of the type of prolapse in complex lesions and is particularly effective in detection or identification of an enterocele or an occult prolapse. MRI staging of prolapse still cannot be used in practice because it is poorly correlated to the clinical examination, which remains the gold standard. In the current state of knowledge, dynamic MRI cannot replace clinical examination and in order to avoid overtreatment a new MRI classification ensuring closer correlation with prolapse symptoms is clearly necessary.

The main contribution of ultrasound still consists in the study of pelvic-perineal meshes and urethral mobility assessment. With three-dimensional reconstructions, it effectively highlights the retraction of meshes. Even if endoanal ultrasound remains the gold standard for exploration of anal sphincter injuries, 3D perineal ultrasound can highlight atrophy or rupture of the anal sphincter while being much less invasive for patients.

The currently available studies have a low level of evidence and there is presently no persuasive proof of the usefulness of imaging in surgical management of urinary incontinence or POP. For the future, the most interesting field of application may reside in detection of levator ani avulsion, which entails exposure to a higher risk of prolapse and surgical repair failure.

References

1. Olsen AL, Smith VJ, Bergstrom JO, Colling JC, Clark AL. Epidemiology of surgically managed pelvic organ prolapse and urinary incontinence. Obstet Gynecol. 1997;89:501–6.
2. Smith FJ, Holman CD, Moorin RE, Tsokos N. Lifetime risk of undergoing surgery for pelvic organ prolapse. Obstet Gynecol. 2010;116:1096–100.
3. Boyles SH, Weber AM, Meyn L. Procedures for pelvic organ prolapse in the United States, 1979–1997. Am J Obstet Gynecol. 2003;188:108–15.
4. Desseauve D, Pierre F, Fritel X. Urinary incontinence in women: study of surgical practice in France. Prog Urol. 2013;23:249–55.
5. Kelvin F, Maglinte DD. Dynamic cystoproctography of female pelvic floor defects and their interrelationships. Am J Roentgenol. 1997;169:769–74.
6. Maglinte DT, Kelvin FM, Fitzgerald K, Hale DS, Benson JT. Association of compartment defects in pelvic floor dysfunction. Am J Roentgenol. 1999;172:439–44.
7. Fritel X, Fauconnier A, Bader G, Cosson M, Debodinance P, Deffieux X, Denys P, Dompeyre P, Faltin D, Fatton B, Haab F, Hermieu JF, Kerdraon J, Mares P, Mellier G, Michel-Laaengh N, Nadeau C, Robain G, de Tayrac R, Jacquetin B. Diagnosis and management of adult female stress urinary incontinence. Guidelines for clinical practice from the French College of Gynaecologists and Obstetricians. Eur J Obstet Gynecol Biol Reprod. 2010;151:14–9.
8. Green TH. Development of a plan for the diagnosis and treatment of urinary stress incontinence. Am J Obstet Gynecol. 1962;83:632–48.
9. Bethoux A, Bory S. Les mécanismes statiques viscéraux pelviens chez la femme à la lumière de l'exploration fonctionnelle du dispositif en position debout. Ann Chir. 1962;16:887–916.
10. Berglas B, Rubin IC. Study of the supportive structures of the uterus by levator myography. Surg Gynecol Obstet. 1953;97:677–92.
11. Sultan AH, Nicholls RJ, Kamm MA, Hudson CN, Beynon J, Bartram CI. Anal endosonography and correlation with in vitro and in vivo anatomy. Br J Surg. 1993;80:508–11.
12. Koelbl H, Bernaschek G, Wolf G. A comparative study of perineal ultrasound scanning and urethrocystography in patients with genuine stress incontinence. Arch Gynecol Obstet. 1988;244:39–45.
13. Yang A, Motstwin J, Rosenheim N, Zerhouni E. Pelvic floor descent in women: dynamic evaluation with fast MR imaging and cinematic display. Radiology. 1991;179:25–33.
14. Johnson JD, Lamensdorf H, Hollander IN, Thurman AE. Use of transvaginale endosonography in the evaluation of women with stress urinary incontinence. J Urol. 1992;147:421–5.
15. Wise BG, Burton G, Cutner A, Cardozo LD. Effect of vaginal ultrasound probe on lower urinary tract function. Br J Urol. 1992;70:12–6.
16. Schaer GN, Schmid T, Peschers U, Delancey JO. Intraurethral ultrasound correlated with urethral histology. Obstet Gynecol. 1998;91:60–4.
17. Koelbl H, Bernaschek G. A new method for sonographic urethrocystography and simultaneous pressure-flow measurements. Obstet Gynecol. 1989;74:417–22.
18. Lee JH, Pretorius DH, Weinstein M, Guaderrama NM, Nager CW, Mittal RK. Transperineal three-dimensional ultrasound in evaluating anal sphincter muscles. Ultrasound Obstet Gynecol. 2007;30:201–9.
19. Yagel S, Valsky DV. Three-dimensional transperineal ultrasonography for evaluation of the anal sphincter complex: another dimension in understanding peripartum sphincter trauma. Ultrasound Obstet Gynecol. 2006;27:119–23.
20. Dietz HP. Ultrasound imaging of the pelvic floor. Part I: two-dimensional aspects. Ultrasound Obstet Gynecol. 2004a;23:80–92.

21. Dietz HP, Wilson PD. Anatomical assessment of the bladder outlet and proximal urethra using ultrasound and video cystourethrography. Int Urogynecol J Pelvic Floor Dysfunct. 1998;9:365–9.
22. Tunn R, Schaer G, Peschers U, Bader W, Gauruder A, Hanzal E, Koelbl H, Koelle D, Perucchini D, Petri E, Riss P, Schuessler B, Viereck V. Updated recommendations on ultrasonography in urogynecology. Int Urogynecol J. 2005;16:236–41.
23. Dietz HP. Ultrasound imaging of the pelvic floor. Part II: three-dimensional or volume imaging. Ultrasound Obstet Gynecol. 2004b;23:615–25.
24. Majida M, Braekken IH, Bø K, Benth JS, Engh ME, Majida M, Braekken IH, Bø K, Benth JS, Engh ME. Validation of three-dimensional perineal ultrasound and magnetic resonance imaging measurements of the pubovisceral muscle at rest. Ultrasound Obstet Gynecol. 2010;35:715–22.
25. Athanasiou S, Khullar V, Boos K, Salvatore S, Cardozo L. Imaging the urethral sphincter with three-dimensional ultrasound. Obstet Gynecol. 1999;94:295–301.
26. Heit M. Intraurethral ultrasonography: correlation of urethral anatomy with functional urodynamic parameters in stress incontinent women. Int Urogynecol J. 2000;11:204–11.
27. Robinson D, Toozs-Hobson P, Cardozo L, Digesu A. Correlating structure and function: three-dimensional ultrasound of the urethral sphincter. Ultrasound Obstet Gynecol. 2004;23:272–6.
28. Oelke M, Mamoulakis C, Ubbink DT, de la Rosette JJ, Wijkstra H. Manual versus automatic bladder wall thickness measurements: a method comparison study. World J Urol. 2009;27:747–53.
29. Oelke M, Khullar V, Wijkstra H. Review on ultrasound measurement of bladder or detrusor wall thickness in women: techniques, diagnostic utility, and use in clinical trials. World J Urol. 2013;31:1093–104.
30. Robinson D, Anders K, Cardozo L, Bidmead J, Toozs-Hobson P, Khullar V. Can ultrasound replace ambulatory urodynamics when investigating women with irritative urinary symptoms? BJOG. 2002;109:145–8.
31. Robinson D, Oelke M, Khullar V, Wijkstra H, Tretter R, Stow B, Compion G, Tubaro A. Bladder wall thickness in women with symptoms of overactive bladder and detrusor overactivity: results from the randomised, placebo-controlled shrink study. Neurourol Urodyn. 2015; doi:10.1002/nau.22808.
32. Frudinger A, Bartram CI, Kamm MA. Transvaginal versus anal endosonography for detecting damage to the anal sphincter. Am J Roentgenol. 1997;168:1435–8.
33. Huang W-C, Yang S-H, Yang J-M. Three-dimensional transperineal sonographic characteristics of the anal sphincter complex in nulliparous women. Ultrasound Obstet Gynecol. 2007;30:210–20.
34. Cornelia L, Stephan B, Michel B, Antoine W, Felix K. Trans-perineal versus endo-anal ultrasound in the detection of anal sphincter tears. Eur J Obstet Gynecol Reprod Biol. 2002;103:79–82.
35. Roos A-M, Abdool Z, Sultan AH, Thakar R. The diagnostic accuracy of endovaginal and transperineal ultrasound for detecting anal sphincter defects: the PREDICT study. Clin Radiol. 2011;66:597–604.
36. Oom DMJ, West RL, Schouten WR, Steensma AB. Detection of anal sphincter defects in female patients with fecal incontinence: a comparison of 3-dimensional transperineal ultrasound and 2-dimensional endoanal ultrasound. Dis Colon Rectum. 2012;55:646–52.
37. Valsky DV, Messing B, Petkova R, Savchev S, Rosenak D, Hochner-Celnikier D, et al. Postpartum evaluation of the anal sphincter by transperineal three-dimensional ultrasound in primiparous women after vaginal delivery and following surgical repair of third-degree tears by the overlapping technique. Ultrasound Obstet Gynecol. 2007;29:195–204.
38. Valsky DV, Cohen SM, Lipschuetz M, Hochner-Celnikier D, Yagel S. Three-dimensional transperineal ultrasound findings associated with anal incontinence after intrapartum sphincter tears in primiparous women. Ultrasound Obstet Gynecol. 2012;39:83–90.

39. Weinstein MM, Pretorius DH, Jung S-A, Nager CW, Mittal RK. Transperineal three-dimensional ultrasound imaging for detection of anatomic defects in the anal sphincter complex muscles. Clin Gastroenterol Hepatol. 2009;7:205–11.
40. Dietz HP, Shek KL, Clarke B. Biometry of the puborectalis muscle and levator hiatus by 3D pelvic floor ultrasound. Ultrasound Obstet Gynecol. 2005;25:580–5.
41. Dietz HP, Wilson PD. Childbirth and pelvic floor trauma. Best Pract Res Clin Obstet Gynaecol. 2005;19:913–24.
42. Van Delft K, Shobeiri SA, Thakar R, Schwertner-Tiepelmann N, Sultan AH. Intra- and interobserver reliability of levator ani muscle biometry and avulsion using three-dimensional endovaginal ultrasonography. Ultrasound Obstet Gynecol. 2014;43:202–9.
43. Peschers U, Schaer G, Anthuber C, Delancey JO, Schuessler B. Changes in vesical neck mobility following vaginal delivery. Obstet Gynecol. 1996;88:1001–6.
44. Dietz HP, Steensma AB, Eldridge A, Grace M, Clarke B. Test-retest and interrater reliability of the ultrasound assessment of bladder neck mobility. In: International Urogynecological Association (IUGA) Conference. 2003: Buenos Aires, Argentina.
45. Brandt FT, Albuquerque CD, Lorenzato FR, Amaral FJ. Perineal assessment of urethrovesical junction mobility in young continent females. Int Urogynecol J. 2000;11:18–22.
46. Bai SW, Chung KA, Rha KH, Kim SU, Kim SK, Park KH. Correlation between urodynamic test results, perineal ultrasound and degree of stress urinary incontinence. J Reprod Med. 2003;48:718–22.
47. Dietz HP, Eldridge A, Grace M, Clarke B. Pelvic organ descent in young nulligravid women. Am J Obstet Gynecol. 2004;191:95–9.
48. Dietz HP, Steensma AB. Posterior compartment prolapse on two-dimensional and three-dimensional pelvic floor ultrasound: the distinction between true rectocele, perineal hypermobility and enterocele. Ultrasound Obstet Gynecol. 2005;26:3–7.
49. Dietz HP, Haylen BT, Broome J. Ultrasound in the quantification of female pelvic organ prolapse. Ultrasound Obstet Gynecol. 2001a;18:511–4.
50. Broekhuis SR, Kluivers KB, Hendriks JC, Fütterer JJ, Barentsz JO, Vierhout ME. POP-Q, dynamic MR imaging, and perineal ultrasonography: do they agree in the quantification of female pelvic organ prolapse? Int Urogynecol J. 2009;20:541–9.
51. Kluivers KB, Hendriks JC, Shek C, Dietz HP. Pelvic organ prolapse symptoms in relation to POPQ, ordinal stages and ultrasound prolapse assessment. Int Urogynecol J. 2008;19:1299–302.
52. Orno AK, Dietz HP. Levator co-activation is a significant confounder of pelvic organ descent on Valsalva maneuver. Ultrasound Obstet Gynecol. 2007;30:346–50.
53. De Leon J, Steensma A, Shek KL, Dietz HP. Ballooning: how to define abnormal distensibility of the levator hiatus. Ultrasound Obstet Gynecol. 2007;30:367–455.
54. Konstantinovic ML, Steensma AB, Domali E, Timmerman D, De Ridder D, Deprest J. Quantification of the pelvic floor contraction using 3D/4D translabial ultrasound. Ultrasound Obstet Gynecol. 2007;30:447–8.
55. Dietz HP, Wilson PD, Clarke B. The use of perineal ultrasound to quantify levator activity and teach pelvic floor muscle exercises. Int Urogynecol J. 2001;12:166–8. discussion 168–9
56. Colaiacomo MC, Masseli G, Polettini I, Lanciotti S, Casciani E, Bertini L, Gualdi G. Dynamic MR imaging of the pelvic floor: a pictorial review. Radiographics. 2009;29:e35.
57. Schoenenberger AW, Debatin JF, Guldenschuh I, Hany TF, Steiner P, Krestin GP. Dynamic MR defecography with a superconducing, open-configuration MR system. Radiology. 1998;206:641–6.
58. Bertschinger KM, Hetzer FH, Roos JE, Treiber K, Marincek B, Hilfiker PR. Dynamic MR imaging of the pelvic floor performed with patient sitting in an open-magnet unit versus with patient supine in a closed-magnet unit. Radiology. 2002;223:501–8.
59. Fauconnier A, Zareski E, Abichedid J, Bader G, Falissard B, Fritel X. Dynamic magnetic resonance imaging for grading pelvic organ prolapse according to international incontinence society classification: which line should be used? Neurourol Urodyn. 2008;27:191–7.

60. Goh V, Halligan S, Kaplan G, Healy JC, Bartram CI. Dynamic MR imaging of the pelvic floor in asymptomatic subjects. Am J Roentgenol. 2000;174:661–6.
61. Lieneman A, Sprenger D, Janssen U, Grosch E, Pellengahr C, Anthuber C. Assessment of pelvic organ by use of functional cine MRI: which reference line should be used? Neurourol Urodyn. 2004;23:3–37.
62. Lakeman MM, Zijta FM, Peringa J, Nederveen AJ, Stoker J, Roovers JP. Dynamic magnetic resonance imaging to quantify pelvic organ prolapse: reliability of assessment and correlation with clinical findings and pelvic floor symptoms. Int Urogynecol J. 2012;23:1547–54.
63. Morren GL, Balasingam AG, Wells JE, Hunter AM, Coates RH, Perry RE. Triphasic MRI of pelvic organ descent: sources of measurement error. Eur J Radiol. 2005;54:276–83.
64. Mortele KJ, Fairhurst J. Dynamic MR defecography of the posterior compartment: indications, techniques and MRI features. Eur J Radiol. 2007;61:462–72.
65. Gousse AE, Barbaric ZL, Safir MH, Madjar S, Marumoto AK, Raz S. Dynamic half Fourier acquisition, single shot turbo spin-echo magnetic resonance imaging for evaluating the female pelvis. J Urol. 2000;164:1606–13.
66. Tunn R, DeLancey JO, Quint EE. Visibility of pelvic organ support system structures in magnetic resonance images without an endovaginal coil. Am J Obstet Gynecol. 2001;184:1156–63.
67. Kelvin FM, Maglinte DD, Hale DS, Benson JT. Female pelvic organ prolapse: a comparison of triphasic dynamic MR imaging and triphasic fluoroscopic cystocolpoproctography. Am J Roentgenol. 2000;174:81–8.
68. Tumbarello JA, Hsu Y, Lewicky-Gaupp C, Rohrer S, De Lancey JO. Do repetitive valsalva maneuvers change maximum prolapse on dynamic MRI? Int Urogynecol J. 2010;21:1247–51.
69. Woodfield CA, Hampton BS, Sung V, Brody JM. Magnetic resonance imaging of pelvic organ prolapse: comparing pubococcygeal and midpubic lines with clinical staging. Int Urogynecol J. 2009;20:695–701.
70. Rouanet JP, Mares P, Courtieu C, Maubon A. L'IRM statique et dynamique du plancher pelvien féminin normal et pathologique [Static and dynamic MRI of the normal and pathological female pelvic floor]. J Gynecol Obstet Biol Reprod. 2000;29:237–41.
71. Bump RC, Mattiasson A, Bø K, Brubaker LP, DeLancey JO, Klarskov P, Shull BL, et al. The standardization of terminology of female pelvic organ prolapse and pelvic floor dysfunction. Am J Obstet Gynecol. 1996;175:10–7.
72. Pannu HK, Kaufman HS, Cundiff GW, Genadry R, Bluemke DA, Fishman EK. Dynamic MR imaging of pelvic organ prolapse: spectrum of abnormalities. Radiographics. 2000;20:1567–82.
73. Healy JC, Halligan S, Reznek RH, Watson S, Bartram CI, Phillips R, Armstrong P. Dynamic MR imaging compared with evacuation proctography when evaluating anorectal configuration and pelvic floor movement. Am J Roentgenol. 1997;169:775–9.
74. Otto SD, Oesterheld A, Ritz JP, Gröne J, Wolf KJ, Buhr HJ, Kroesen A. Rectal anatomy after rectopexy: cinedefecography versus MR-defecography. J Surg Res. 2011;165:52–8.
75. Dvorkin LS, Hetzer F, Scott SM, Williams NS, Gedroye W, Luniss PJ. Open-magnet MR defaecography compared with evacuation proctography in the diagnosis and management of patients with rectal intussusception. Color Dis. 2004;6:45–53.
76. Foti PV, Farina R, Riva G, Coronella M, Fisichella E, Palmucci S, Racalbuto A, Politi G, Ettorre GC. Pelvic floor imaging: comparison between magnetic resonance imaging and conventional defecography in studying outlet obstruction syndrome. Radiol Med. 2013;118:23–39.
77. Strohbehn K, Ellis JH, Strohbehn JA, DeLancey JO. Magnetic resonance imaging of the levator ani with anatomic correlation. Obstet Gynecol. 1996;87:277–85.
78. Rouanet JP, de Graef M, Mares P, Maubon A. IRM du plancher pelvien de la jeune femme nullipare du normal à l'anormal. in Séminaire scientifique gynécologique. J Fr Radiol. 2004;44:173–86.

79. Fauconnier A, Delmas V, Lassau JP, Boccon-Gibod L. Ventral tethering of the vagina and its role in the kinetics of urethra and bladder-neck straining. Surg Radiol Anat. 1996;18:81–7.
80. Hjartardóttir S, Nilsson J, Petersen C, Lingman G. The female pelvic floor: a dome – not a basin. Acta Obstet Gynecol Scand. 1997;76:567–71.
81. Singh K, Reid WM, Berger LA. Assessment and grading of pelvic organ prolapse by use of dynamic magnetic resonance imaging. Am J Obstet Gynecol. 2001;185:71–7.
82. Yoshioka K, Matsui Y, Yamada O, Sakaguchi M, Takada H, Hioki K, Yamamoto M, et al. Physiologic and anatomic assessment of patients with rectocele. Dis Colon Rectum. 1991;34:704–8.
83. Comiter CV, Vasavada SP, Barbaric ZL, Gousse AE, Raz s. Grading pelvic prolapse and pelvic floor relaxation using dynamic magnetic resonance imaging. Urology. 1999;54:454–7.
84. Lammers K, Kluivers KB, Vierhout ME, Prokop M, Fütterer JJ. Inter- and intraobserver reliability for diagnosing levator ani changes on magnetic resonance imaging. Ultrasound Obstet Gynecol. 2013;42:347–52.
85. Dietz HP, Clarke B, Herbison B. Bladder neck mobility and urethral closure pressure as predictors of genuine stress incontinence. Int Urogynecol J. 2002;13:289–93.
86. Pregazzi R, Sartore A, Bortoli P, Grimaldi E, Troiano L, Guaschino S. Perineal ultrasound evaluation of urethral angle and bladder neck mobility in women with stress urinary incontinence. BJOG. 2002;109:821–7.
87. Dietz HP, Clarke B. The urethral pressure profile and ultrasound imaging of the lower urinary tract. Int Urogynecol J. 2001;12:38–41.
88. Huang WC, Yang JM. Bladder neck funneling on ultrasound cystourethrography in primary stress urinary incontinence: a sign associated with urethral hypermobility and intrinsic sphincter deficiency. Urology. 2003;61:936–41.
89. Schaer GN, Perucchini D, Munz E, Peschers U, Koechli OR, Delancey JO. Sonographic evaluation of the bladder neck in continent and stress-incontinent women. Obstet Gynecol. 1999;93:412–6.
90. Kim JK, Kim YJ, Choo MS, Cho KS. The urethra and its supporting structures in women with stress urinary incontinence: MR imaging using an endovaginal coil. Am J Roentgenol. 2003;180:1037–44.
91. Tunn R, Paris S, Fischer W, Hamm B, Kuchinke J. Static magnetic resonance imaging of the pelvic floor muscle morphology in women with stress urinary incontinence and pelvic prolapse. Neurourol Urodyn. 1998;17:579–89.
92. Fritel X, Zabak K, Pigné A, Demaria F, Bénifla JL. Predictive value of urethra mobility before sub-urethra tape procedure for urinary stress incontinence in women. J Urol. 2002;168:2472–5.
93. Cortes E, Reid WM, Singh K, Berger L. Clinical examination and dynamic magnetic resonance imaging in vaginal vault prolapse. Obstet Gynecol. 2004;103:41–6.
94. Broekhuis SR, Kluivers KB, Hendriks JC, Vierhout ME, Barentsz JO, Fütterer JJ. Dynamic magnetic resonance imaging: reliability of anatomical landmarks and reference lines used to assess pelvic organ prolapse. Int Urogynecol J. 2009;20:141–8.
95. Novellas S, Mondot L, Bafghi A, Fournol M, Baudin G, Coco L, Bongain A, Chevallier P. Evaluation of two classifications systems for pelvic prolapse on dynamic MRI. J Radiol. 2009;90:1717–24.
96. Lone FW, Thakar R, Sultan AH, Stankiewicz A. Accuracy of assessing pelvic organ prolapse quantification points using dynamic 2D transperineal ultrasound in women with pelvic organ prolapse. Int Urogynecol J. 2012;23:1555–60.
97. Broekhuis SR, Fütterer JJ, Hendriks JC, Barentsz JO, Vierhout ME, Kluivers KB. Symptoms of pelvic floor dysfunction are poorly correlated with findings on clinical examination and dynamic MR imaging of the pelvic floor. Int Urogynecol J. 2009c;20:1169–74.
98. Kearney R, Miller JM, Ashton-Miller JA, DeLancey JO. Obstetric factors associated with levatorani muscle injury after vaginal birth. Obstet Gynecol. 2006;107:144–9.

99. Abdool Z, Shek KL, Dietz HP. The effect of levator avulsion on hiatal dimension and function. Am J Obstet Gynecol. 2009;201:89 e1–5.
100. Billecocq S, Morel MP, Fritel X. Traumatismes du levator ani après l'accouchement, de l'étirement à l'avulsion: revue de la littérature [Levator ani trauma after childbirth, from stretch injury to avulsion: review of the literature]. Prog Urol. 2013;23:511–8.
101. DeLancey JO, Morgan DM, Fenner DE, Kearney R, Guire K, Miller JM, Hussain H, et al. Comparison of levator ani muscle defects and function in women with and without pelvic organ prolapse. Obstet Gynecol. 2007;109:295–302.
102. Chen L, Ashton-Miller JA, DeLancey JO. A 3D finite element model of anterior vaginal wall support to evaluate mechanisms underlying cystocele formation. J Biomech. 2009;42:1371–7.
103. Dietz HP, Steensma AB. The prevalence of major abnormalities of the levator ani in urogynaecological patients. BJOG. 2006;113:225–30.
104. Heilbrun M, Nygaard I, Lockhart M, Richter H, Brown M, Kenton K, et al. Correlation between levator ani muscle injuries on MRI and fecal incontinence, pelvic organ prolapse and urinary incontinence in primiparous women. Int Urogynecol J. 2009;20:967–72.
105. Morgan DM, Cardoza P, Guire K, Fenner DE, DeLancey JO. Levator ani defect status and lower urinary tract symptoms in women with pelvic organ prolapse. Int Urogynecol J. 2010;21:47–52.
106. Brincat CA, Delancey JO, Miller LM. Urethral closure pressures among primiparous women with and without levator ani muscle defects. Int Urogynecol J. 2011;22:1491–5.
107. Bernstein IT. The pelvic floor muscles: muscle thickness in healthy and urinary-incontinent women measured by perineal ultrasonography with reference to the effect of pelvic floor training. Estrogen receptor studies. Neurourol Urodyn. 1997;16:237–75.
108. Lehur PA, Leroi AM. Incontinence anale de l'adulte: recommandations pour la pratique clinique [Anal incontinence in the adult: recommendations for clinical practice]. Ann Chir. 2000;125:511–21.
109. Deen KI, Kumar D, Williams JG, Olliff J, Keighley MR. Anal sphincter defects. Correlation between endoanal ultrasound and surgery. Ann Surg. 1993;218:201–5.
110. Sultan AH, Kamm MA, Talbot IC, Nicholls RJ, Bartram CI. Anal endosonography for identifying external sphincter defects confirmed histologically. Br J Surg. 1994;81:463–5.
111. Starck M, Bohe M, Valentin L. Results of endosonographic imaging of the anal sphincter 2-7 days after primary repair of third- or fourth-degree obstetric sphincter tears. Ultrasound Obstet Gynecol. 2003;22:609–15.
112. Starck M, Bohe M, Valentin L. The extent of endosonographic anal sphincter defects after primary repair of obstetric sphincter tears increases over time and is related to anal incontinence. Ultrasound Obstet Gynecol. 2006;27:188–97.
113. Sentovich SM, Blatchford GJ, Rivela LJ, Lin K, Thorson AG, Christensen MA. Diagnosing anal sphincter injury with transanal ultrasound and manometry. Dis Colon Rectum. 1997;40:1430–4.
114. Williams AB, Bartram CI, Halligan S, Spencer JA, Nicholls RJ, Kmiot WA. Anal sphincter damage after vaginal delivery using three-dimensional endosonography. Obstet Gynecol. 2001;97:770–5.
115. Fletcher JG, Busse RF, Riederer SJ, Hough D, Gluecker T, Harper CM, Bharucha AE. Magnetic resonance imaging of anatomic and dynamic defects of the pelvic floor in defecatory disorders. Am J Gastroenterol. 2003;98:399–411.
116. Rociu E, Stoker J, Eijkemans MJ, Schouten WR, Laméris JS. Fecal incontinence: endoanal US versus endoanal MR imaging. Radiology. 1999;212:453–8.
117. Terra MP, Beets-Tan RG, van Der Hulst VP, Dijkgraaf MG, Bossuyt PM, Dobben AC, Baeten CG, Stoker J. Anal sphincter defects in patients with fecal incontinence: endoanal versus external phased-array MR imaging. Radiology. 2005;236:886–95.

118. Cazemier M et al. Atrophy and defects detection of the external anal sphincter: comparison between three-dimensional anal endosonography and endoanal magnetic resonance imaging. Dis Colon Rectum. 2006;49:20–7.
119. Faltin DL, Boulvain M, Irion O, Bretones S, Stan C, Weil A. Diagnosis of anal sphincter tears by postpartum endosonography to predict fecal incontinence. Obstet Gynecol. 2000;95:643–7.
120. Timor-Tritsch IE, Monteagudo A, Smilen SW, Porges RF, Référence Avizova E. Simple ultrasound evaluation of the anal sphincter in female patients using a transvaginal transducer. Ultrasound Obstet Gynecol. 2005;25:177–83.
121. Maslovitz S, Jaffa A, Levin I, Almog B, Lessing JB, Wolman I. The clinical significance of postpartum transperineal ultrasound of the anal sphincter. Eur J Obstet Gynecol Reprod Biol. 2007;134:115–9.
122. Hetzer FH, Andreseik GA, Tsagari C, Sahrbacher U, Weishaupt D. MR defecography in patients with fecal incontinence: imaging findings and their effects on surgical management. Radiology. 2006;240:449–57.
123. Viereck V, Pauer HU, Hesse O, Bader W, Tunn R, Lange R, Hilgers R, Emons G. Urethral hypermobility after anti-incontinence surgery – a prognostic indicator? Int Urogynecol J. 2006;17:586–92.
124. Martan A, Masata J, Halaska M, Voigt R. Ultrasound imaging of the lower urinary system in women after Burch colposuspension. Ultrasound Obstet Gynecol. 2001;17:58–64.
125. Sarlos D, Kuronen M, Schaer GN. How does tension-free vaginal tape correct stress incontinence? Investigation by perineal ultrasound. Int Urogynecol J. 2003;14:395–8.
126. Masata J, Masata J, Martan A, Svabik K, Drahoradova P, Pavlikova M. Ultrasound imaging of the lower urinary tract after successful tension-free vaginal tape (TVT) procedure. Ultrasound Obstet Gynecol. 2006;28:221–8.
127. Ducarme G, Rey D, Ménard Y, Staerman F. Echographie endovaginale et troubles mictionnels après TVT [Transvaginal ultrasound and voiding disorders after TVT procedure]. Gynecol Obstet Fertil. 2004;32:18–22.
128. Lammers K, Fütterer JJ, Prokop M, Vierhout ME, Kluivers KB. Diagnosing pubovisceral avulsions: a systematic review of the clinical relevance of a prevalent anatomical defect. Int Urogynecol J. 2012;23:1653–64.
129. Morgan DM, Larson K, Lewicky-Gaupp C, Fenner DE, Delancey JO. Vaginal support as determined by levatorani defect status 6 weeks after primary surgery for pelvic organ prolapse. Int J Gynaecol Obstet. 2011;114:141–4.
130. Weemhoff M, Vergeldt TF, Notten K, Serroyen J, Kampschoer PH, Roumzn FJ. Avulsion of puborectalis muscle and other risk factors for cystocele recurrence: a 2-year follow-up study. Int Urogynecol J. 2012;23:65–71.
131. Schuettoff S, Beyersdorff D, Gauruder-Burmester A, Tunn R. Visibility of the polypropylene tape after tension-free vaginal tape (TVT) procedure in women with stress urinary incontinence: comparison of introital ultrasound and magnetic resonance imaging in vitro and in vivo. Ultrasound Obstet Gynecol. 2006;27:687–92.
132. Tunn R, Picot A, Marschke J, Gauruder-Burmester A. Sonomorphological evaluation of polypropylene mesh implants after vaginal mesh repair in women with cystocele or rectocele. Ultrasound Obstet Gynecol. 2007;29:449–52.
133. Letouzey V, et al. Etude de la rétraction prothétique dans la cure de prolapsus voie basse par échographie périnéale. In: XXXIIème congrès de la SIFUD. 2009, Marseille.

Chapter 8
Perineal Trauma and Its Impact on Women's Health

Sara Webb, Katariina Laine, and Jan Willem de Leeuw

Abstract Giving birth is one of the major positive life events in a woman's life. In the vast majority of women, vaginal delivery is not associated with direct complications or consequences for her health in later life. However, in some women childbirth impacts on both the physical and psychological health of a woman. Injury to the pelvic floor can occur through direct perineal trauma, damage to the pelvic floor muscles and connective tissues and pelvic nerve injury. The majority of women who sustain perineal trauma during childbirth as long as it repaired appropriately and provided with good postnatal care, will heal reasonably quickly with no long-term morbidity. However, complications can occur that lead to problems at the short or even the longer term. Such complications include, infection, wound dehiscence, granulation tissue formation, pain, sexual dysfunction as well as urinary and bowel problems, e.g. urinary retention and incontinence and anal incontinence. This chapter aims to provide health care professionals caring for women with childbirth-related perineal trauma with an insight into such complications and their consequences hence enabling them to provide timely interventions to mitigate such risks.

Keywords Perineal injury • Anal incontinence • Urinary incontinence • Perineal pain • Pelvic floor

S. Webb (✉)
Birmingham Women's NHS Foundation Trust, Birmingham, UK
e-mail: sara.webb@bwnft.nhs.uk

K. Laine
Oslo University Hospital, Ullevål, Norway
e-mail: kattiksen@yahoo.no

J.W. de Leeuw
Ikazia Hospital, Rotterdam, The Netherlands
e-mail: jw.de.leeuw@ikazia.nl

K.M.K. Ismail (ed.), *Perineal Trauma at Childbirth*,
DOI 10.1007/978-3-319-14860-1_8

Introduction

Childbirth is one of the major life events for a woman and should be considered as a normal physiological phenomenon without major health consequences for the vast majority of women. There is, however, a group of women that may suffer physical or psychological, or both, health problems after giving birth. Gyhagen et al. [1] have shown in a large postal questionnaire study from Sweden that 20 years after one vaginal delivery just under 50 % of women reported one or more pelvic floor disorder (PFD) (i.e. urinary of faecal incontinence or pelvic organ prolapse). Compared to women who had delivered by caesarean section the risk of this type of complaints was significantly increased. These findings corroborate the results from the PROLONG study group who showed that complaints of PFD are common after vaginal delivery and are associated with various modes of delivery. However, both the Swedish study and the studies from the UK have shown that these complaints cannot be prevented by delivering by caesarean section exclusively, suggesting that pregnancy itself and other non-obstetrical factors are involved too [2–5]. Furthermore, these studies have investigated the association of delivery with PFD's but did not investigate a possible role of perineal trauma itself in the advent of PFD's.

Injury to the pelvic floor can occur through direct perineal trauma, damage to the pelvic floor muscles and connective tissues, and pelvic nerve injury. Perineal trauma resulting from vaginal delivery is common and affects millions of women every year. Worldwide differences in reporting practices and definitions result in a wide variation of reported childbirth related perineal trauma rates between individual countries [6]. In the UK up to 80 % of women delivering their first child need suturing of the perineal area, resulting from a spontaneous tear and/or an episiotomy [7]. The majority of women who sustain perineal trauma during childbirth, if repaired appropriately and provided with good postnatal care, will usually heal reasonably quickly with no long-term morbidity [8]. However, in some women complications may arise, such as infection, wound dehiscence, scar tissue formation, areas of overgranulated tissue. This may lead to longer term morbidity such as persistent pain, dyspareunia, urinary and bowel symptoms and even fistulae that can have serious detrimental effects on their physical, psychosocial and sexual wellbeing [9, 10]. This chapter aims to provide health care professionals caring for women with perineal trauma in the postnatal period an understanding of the possible short and long term complications that may occur and management options as well as provide advice and support for affected women.

Infection

Fear of perineal injury requiring stitches and worry about infection and wound breakdown consistently remains a priority concern for women, worldwide [11, 12]. Perkins et al. identified that for women in both the UK and in Brazil, who had sustained childbirth related perineal trauma, fear of a perineal infection remained as either the first or one of the top four concerns at regular intervals throughout the first 3 months postpartum [13]. Despite this being a major concern for childbearing women there is no standard universal definition of childbirth related perineal wound infection. There is also a lack of information as to the exact rates of such infection and wound dehiscence. Rates of less than 2 % are common but rates of up to 20 %, depending on the type of perineal trauma studied, are reported [14, 15]. Indeed, this data is difficult to capture accurately due to lack of integrated technology systems linking primary, secondary and community services [12]. Therefore, it is impossible to give any reliable estimate of the these rates.

There are many factors that may contribute to delay in wound healing that include operative vaginal delivery, smoking, underlying medical conditions, obesity, stress, malnutrition, poor primary repair resulting from inappropriate methods and/or materials and misdiagnosis of extent of trauma [15–19]. Therefore, it is vital that women falling into any of these high risk categories are aware of such risk and provided with how to reduce it and who to contact if they had any concerns.

In general, women should be offered examination of the perineum at each postnatal visit by the midwife or GP and any signs/symptoms should be acted on promptly to reduce any risk of infection leading to wound dehiscence [8]. The REEDA wound assessment scoring tool (Table 8.1) was designed to facilitate measurement of healing of an episiotomy using five components of the healing process that t may suggest infection such as increase in pain, oedema, excessive/offensive discharge, feeling unwell, pyrexia, wound dehiscence or abscess formation [20]. The REEDA scoring proved valuable with students as a method of increasing their observational skills for perineal wound healing complications and assisting with reducing associated pain during the postnatal period. However, a more recent study has demonstrated the REEDA tool has poor inter-rater reliability on some components and needs further enhancement [21]. This suggests that this scale may be helpful in the individual patient when used by one physician or midwife during follow-up of the healing process, but care should be taken with the interpretation when comparing assessments of different observators.

If infection is suspected a wound swab should be taken to identify causative organisms and a broad spectrum (including anaerobes) antibiotic prescribed. It has been shown that routine swabbing in the absence of any clinical signs of infection is not cost-effective and only likely to reveal non-causative bacteria and flora [22].

Wound Dehiscence

As with infection, wound dehiscence is relatively rare. Wound dehiscence, either partial (opening of skin and/or vaginal wall and/or superficial perineal muscles) or complete (opening of the skin, vaginal wall, superficial and deep muscle layers), is, if occurring, frequently reported to be a consequence of infection. Current practice

Table 8.1 The REEDA wound assessment tool [18]

Score	Redness	Edema	Ecchymosis (Bruising)	Discharge	Approximation
0	None	None	None	None	Closed
1	Mild	Mild	Mild	Serum	Skin separation 3 mm or less
	Less than 0.5 cm from each side of the wound edges	Less than 1 cm from each side of the wound edges	Less than 1 cm from each side of the wound edges		
2	Moderate	Moderate	Moderate	Serosanguinous	Skin and subcutaneous fat separation
	0.5–1 cm from each side of the wound edges	1–2 cm from each side of the wound edges	1–2 cm from each side of the wound edges		
3	Severe	Severe	Severe	Purulent	Skin and subcutaneous fat and fascial layer separation
	More than 1 cm from each side of the wound edges	More than 2 cm from each side of the wound edges	More than 2 cm from each side of the wound edges		
Total					

favours expectant management with antibiotic cover and allowing the dehisced wound to heal with secondary intention. This is a protracted process whereby granulation tissue fills the open space between the skin edges. An alternative option is for admission to hospital and re-suturing of the wound following debridement of the wound edges. A Cochrane systematic review shows that there is currently no high level evidence to support the promotion of either management option [23]. In response, a randomised-controlled-trial (RCT) has been undertaken to establish the feasibility of conducting a full-scale RCT to evaluate the effectiveness of both options, but results of this first study addressing this phenomenon have to be awaited [24]. Regardless of the management option chosen, it is imperative that women with perineal infection are reviewed as a matter of urgency, prescribed the most appropriate antibiotic and they are regularly monitored throughout the healing process. Although the absolute numbers are small, perineal wound infection was identified as a cause of systemic sepsis and mortality illustrating the need for early identification, effective management and careful follow up [25].

Excessive Granulation Tissue

Perineal wounds, healing by either primary or secondary intention, may develop excessive granulation tissue, sometimes referred to as 'over healed tissue'. More collagen is produced when healing is protracted which can lead to an increase in areas of over-granulated tissue, scarring, tissue flexibility and further infection.

Areas of over-granulated tissue can become very sore and women often complain of what they perceive to be a skin tag that bleeds on contact and can produce excessive discharge. In the majority of cases these areas of tissue resolve spontaneously over time. Occasionally they may need removal with topical application of silver nitrate to 'dissolve' the tissue, which can be performed in an outpatient setting. However, if the area is too large this may need excision under local or regional anaesthesia. Excessive scar tissue or poor alignment of tissues either from poor initial repair or as a result of wound dehiscence may require future corrective surgery, such as modified Fenton's procedure, perineal refashioning or perineorrhaphy [26].

Perineal Pain and Sexual Function

Perineal pain, dyspareunia and impaired sexual drive can continue for many years after childbirth [27–29]. In a prospective cohort study from the UK 92 % of women experienced perineal pain on the first day after delivery, but in almost 90 % of these women, this resolved within 2 months [30]. In this cohort OASIS appeared to be the most painful type of perineal trauma, whereas mediolateral episiotomies were more painful than spontaneous second degree tears. An observational study from Norway showed that on the first day after delivery only less than 20 % of women reported pain VAS-scores of 7 or higher (on a scale of 0–10). Furthermore, in contrast to the general belief, there was no significant difference in perineal pain between midline, mediolateral or lateral episiotomies on the first day after delivery [31].

In daily practice, immediately after delivery, perineal pain in the absence of hematoma or infection is treated conservatively with rest, ice packs and oral paracetamol.

In a large prospective cohort study from Australia, 83 % of women had resumed vaginal intercourse by 18 months postpartum. Of these women 24 % reported dyspareunia. In this study, sutured spontaneous perineal tears or episiotomies were not independently associated with dyspareunia 18 months after delivery (Adj OR: 1.37, 95 % CI: 0.8–2.2) [32].

In a large Norwegian study using postal questionnaires more than 50 % of the responders had resumed intercourse 8 weeks after delivery, increasing to 75 % at 12 weeks and almost 95 % 1 year after delivery [33]. In this study the odds for postponing the first intercourse after delivery were more than five times higher for women after OASIS compared to women with an intact perineum (Adj OR: 5.52, 95 % CI: 1.59–19.16). All other types of perineal trauma were not significantly associated with postponement of first intercourse after delivery.

OASI was also the only significant predictor for dyspareunia 1 year after delivery (Adj OR: 3.57, 95 % CI: 1.39–9.19). Again episiotomy was not associated with dyspareunia 1 year after delivery.

Van Brummen et al. showed in their prospective study from the Netherlands that women were five times less likely to be sexually active 1 year after delivery after a third/fourth degree anal sphincter tear as compared with women with an intact perineum (Adj OR: 0.2, 95 % CI: 0.04–0.93) [34]. In this study dissatisfaction with the sexual relationship 1 year after childbirth was significantly associated with being sexually active at 12 weeks of gestation and older maternal age at delivery, suggesting that sexual satisfaction after deliver may be more related to other pregnancy- and parturition-associated factors.

These findings are in contrast with earlier studies that showed that women with an intact perineum (compared with those who have experienced perineal trauma) are more likely to resume intercourse earlier, report less pain with first sexual intercourse, report greater satisfaction with sexual experience and report greater sexual sensation and likelihood of orgasm at 6 months postpartum [35–37]. Whether these different outcomes are associated with newer techniques and materials for the repair of perineal trauma or other factors remains unclear.

Women often wait for review by their physician or midwife prior to commencing sexual intercourse for reassurance that it is safe to do so and that all trauma has fully healed [35]. Although it is not certain that perineal trauma in general affects the resumption of sexual function, clinicians should be aware in the period after delivery that childbirth can affect sexual function through many ways, such as physical damage to the perineal tissues, pudendal neuropathy, vaginal dryness resultant from hormonal changes, alterations in lifestyle and the presence of a baby in the family [28]. Nevertheless, it is important that clinicians caring for all postnatal women, regardless of extent of perineal trauma, discuss postpartum sexual function, possible changes and give advice and guidance. Women need to be reassured that changes to sexual function and desire is normal and that the majority of women do not report significant changes at the long term.

However, women should be advised that if dyspareunia continues to be an ongoing problem, early referral to a specialist should be requested as this generally persists [38]. Persistent perineal pain and/or dyspareunia may be the long term consequence of excessive scar tissue or poor alignment of tissues which may require reconstructive surgery [26, 27]. Fodstad et al. and Stedenfeldt et al. showed that persisting sexual problems, including dyspareunia, are associated with larger perineal trauma, i.e. OASIS [33, 39]. Mous et al. described in their retrospective cohort study that even after 25 years 29 % of women who sustained an OASIS reported dyspareunia, compared to 13 % of controls (women with first or second degree perineal tear or mediolateral episiotomy) [27].

These studies show that even if dyspareunia persists after delivery, women may be reluctant to report this directly to their clinician. An open attitude of clinicians with the ability to enquire with empathy is therefore very important. Depending on the severity of the symptoms and extent of the eventually necessary corrective surgery required, this may impact on the mode of future births. Nevertheless, this is an informed decision that women should be supported to make in order to prevent long term physical, psychological and relationship issues.

Bladder and Bowel Dysfunction

Bladder and bowel dysfunction may a have serious effect on the quality of life of both men and women. In women, pregnancy and childbirth in itself is associated with these complaints, but the exact role of perineal injury in the advent of these complaints is studied less extensively [2–5, 40]. In this paragraph, the association of perineal injury with different types of bladder and bowel dysfunction is highlighted.

Bladder Symptoms

Due to anatomical and physiological changes urinary symptoms are common in pregnancy. However, these may become permanent due to nerve and tissue damage resulting from labour and the birth. Bladder symptoms as urinary incontinence and voiding difficulties such as hesitancy and urinary retention are associated with first labour, instrumental delivery, long labour and epidural [41–43].

In the immediate postpartum period urinary retention may occur. Overt urinary retention in the postpartum period (PUR), i.e. the inability to void spontaneously within 6 h of vaginal birth or removal of a catheter after a caesarean section, is reported in 0.3–4.7 % of women [44]. In a recent meta-analysis, PUR was significantly associated with episiotomy (OR 4.8, 95 % CI: 2.0–12.0). Although this suggests that perineal trauma is an important causative factor, one must realise that other obstetrical factors, e.g. operative vaginal delivery, epidural analgesia and primiparity, are also significantly associated with PUR [45]. Therefore, although not necessarily a direct complication of perineal trauma, these women may well be experiencing bladder symptoms in the postnatal period. The pain and discomfort of which may be intensified due to the nature and location of the trauma, such as paraurethral tears and anterior labial grazes and lacerations. Women need to be reassured that such bladder function changes following birth are common and given voiding advice to help both minimise short term pain during micturition and avoid long term bladder damage.

Vaginal childbirth itself is associated with an increased risk of urinary incontinence (UI) in later life [46]. In a large Norwegian cohort study Rortveit et al. showed that 57 % of UI among women with one vaginal birth and 64 % of UI among women with two vaginal births can be attributed to vaginal delivery itself when comparing these women to nulliparous controls [47]. In this study a vaginal birth was associated with stress and mixed urinary incontinence but not with urge urinary incontinence. Furthermore, this association existed only for women up to the age of 50 years. MacArtur et al. described the results of a prospective cohort study with a 12 year follow-up and showed that UI was associated with vaginal birth, with operative vaginal birth carrying the same risk as spontaneous delivery [4]. Compared with having only spontaneous vaginal deliveries (SVDs), women who delivered exclusively by caesarean section were less likely to have persistent UI (Adj. OR 0.42, 95 % CI 0.33–0.54). Unfortunately, both these studies did not address the relation of perineal trauma itself with UI in later life.

In a large cohort study from the United States, urinary incontinence 5–10 years after the first vaginal delivery appeared to occur independently of any type of perineal trauma, even if perineal trauma had occurred more than once [48]. Studies addressing the possible association of UI with higher degrees of perineal trauma, i.e. OASIS, showed no relation between OASIS and UI in later life, although shortly after delivery UI may be more common in women with OASIS [49]. It appears that in women with OASIS, as in women with a vaginal delivery with lower degrees or no perineal trauma, "age is the great equalizer" with regard to the occurrence of urinary incontinence.

Bowel Symptoms

Vaginal birth is considered to be the most important moment in the advent of anal incontinence (AI) in women [9]. Historically the definition of AI has been limited to the involuntary loss of faces [50]. However, the more recent definition from the International Continence Society states that 'Anal incontinence is the involuntary loss of flatus, liquid or solid stool that is a social or hygienic problem' includes symptoms of urgency and flatus incontinence and, equally importantly, the impact of these symptoms on the woman [51]. Despite it being a distressing and disabling condition that has a known negative effect on a woman's quality of life and mental health, it is under reported due to feelings of embarrassment and therefore an under recognised condition [49, 52–54].

The prevalence of defecatory symptoms is two to three times higher for women who sustain an obstetric anal sphincter injury (OASIS) (47–61 %) in comparison to women without (13–22 %) [27, 55, 56]. Sultan et al. were one of the first groups to show that complaints of anal incontinence 7 weeks after delivery are strongly associated with OASIS [55]. A large follow-up study from the Netherlands showed comparable figures with 40 % of women having flatus incontinence 25 years after delivery compared with 10 % of controls [27]. In this study 16 % of women were incontinent for liquid or solid stools after OASIS compared to 5 % of controls. The latter study showed also that the prevalence of these complaints in women with OASIS had significantly risen more than 15 years after delivery. Fifteen years after the index delivery 38 % of women with OASIS reported defecatory symptoms, whereas 10 years later 61 % of these women reported these symptoms. In the control group these numbers were 16 % and 22 % respectively. In both studies anal incontinence was associated with persisting defects of anal sphincter complex despite primary repair immediately after delivery.

Evidence from the literature shows that instrumental delivery, especially forceps delivery, prolonged second stages of labour and infant birth weight >4,000 g are all independent risk factors for AI regardless of the degree of perineal trauma sustained [3, 57–59]. These associations suggest that the direct anatomical damage to the anal sphincters is not the only isolated causative factor for development of AI.

More recent studies have shown that the association of OASIS, especially if persisting sphincter defects are present, with complaints of AI still exists, despite the growing attention for adequate training in repair of OASIS [60–63]. This implies that primary prevention of OASIS during delivery is probably the strongest preventive measure for anal incontinence in women.

However, if anal incontinence is encountered after delivery, every patient deserves proper analysis, examination and the best possible treatment of this embarrassing and socially debilitating condition. Therefore, referral to a centre specialized in the treatment of anal incontinence should be considered. It is to be preferred to refer the patient to a centre that is able to offer all types of treatment, both conservative and surgical [64, 65].

Haemorrhoids and anal fissures are common during the last trimester of pregnancy and within the first month following the birth with constipation identified as the single independent preventable risk factor [66]. For women with perineal trauma the location of the perineal wound may increase pain and discomfort in the postnatal period. Women need to be reassured that such changes following birth are common and encourage women to avoid constipation and straining. As well as being recommended for women with OASIS, the use of stool softeners and bulking agents should be considered for women with lesser degrees of perineal trauma to avoid straining and constipation, as passing hard stools can disrupt the repair [67].

Psychological Aspects

Childbirth related perineal trauma can have a negative impact on a woman's sexuality, self-identity and confidence. This can lead to longer term postnatal depression and impact on her relationship with their partners, family and friends [68]. Research has shown that unexpected injury during pregnancy and childbirth, such as perineal trauma and its associated complications can result in a more stressful period that can result in some women feeling isolated and devalued [69–71]. Women often feel too embarrassed to discuss intimate problems with their partners and family for fear of rejection or being perceived as not fulfilling their role as a woman and wife [72, 73]. It is important that midwives and doctors caring for women in the postnatal period remain supportive and discuss these sensitive issues with women. This will help women overcome feelings of isolation, shame and embarrassment and help women regain their self-confidence as women, partners and mothers.

Fear of Next Pregnancy and Delivery

Some women who experience severe perineal trauma or associated complications can feel frightened and anxious about future pregnancies and births [68, 70, 73]. This can be due to lack of information women received both about the trauma sustained and the detrimental impact pain and discomfort could have in the early postnatal period [73, 74]. This places a great deal of stress on women who are placed in a paradox between the fear of a repeat of the trauma previously experienced, both physical and psychological, and feelings of empowerment and fulfilment of 'achieving a vaginal birth' [73]. Midwives and obstetricians should ensure women are given comprehensive, understandable information about the extent of the perineal trauma, repair, ongoing care and possible complications that arise as this may alleviate any fears and anxieties regarding future pregnancies [68].

Financial Implications

Prolonged healing, associated pain and bladder and bowel symptoms associated with complications of perineal trauma can have financial implications. Women may delay returning to employment due to prolonged perineal pain affecting their ability to mobilise or complete everyday duties [74, 75]. Not only may returning to work be delayed, women may even sometimes stop working due to the constraints placed by bowel and bladder urgency and incontinence [76].

Summary

Although childbirth is generally considered to be a positive life event, childbirth related perineal trauma may have an impact on both the physical and psychological health in a selected group of women and their families that can extend into the longer term. In the immediate postpartum period attention should be paid to ensure optimal wound healing and proper functioning of bladder and bowel. Apart from the focus on the birth and caring for the baby health care professionals should be aware of other issues and complaints related to sexual health and urinary or anal incontinence, especially in women with a history of OASIS.

Hence, it is vital that health professionals caring for women with perineal trauma take a holistic approach where the physical symptoms are managed in conjunction with psychological considerations. It is imperative that well-being of the mother remains a priority and does not become a secondary consideration to that of the baby [77].

References

1. Gyhagen M, Åkervall S, Milsom I. Clustering of pelvic floor disorders 20 years after one vaginal or one cesarean birth. Int Urogynecol J. 2015;26(8):1115–21.
2. Glazener C, Elders A, Macarthur C, Lancashire RJ, Herbison P, Hagen S, Dean N, Bain C, Toozs-Hobson P, Richardson K, McDonald A, McPherson G, Wilson D, ProLong Study Group. Childbirth and prolapse: long-term associations with the symptoms and objective measurement of pelvic organ prolapse. BJOG. 2013;120(2):161–8.
3. MacArthur C, Wilson D, Herbison P, Lancashire RJ, Hagen S, Toozs-Hobson P, Dean N, Glazener C; ProLong study group. Faecal incontinence persisting after childbirth: a 12 year longitudinal study. BJOG. 2013;120(2):169–78.

4. MacArthur C, Wilson D, Herbison P, Lancashire RJ, Hagen S, Toozs-Hobson P, Dean N, Glazener C, Prolong study group. Urinary incontinence persisting after childbirth: extent, delivery history, and effects in a 12-year longitudinal cohort study. BJOG. 2016;123(6):1022–9.
5. Glazener CM, MacArthur C, Hagen S, Elders A, Lancashire R, Herbison GP, Wilson PD, ProLong Study Group. Twelve-year follow-up of conservative management of postnatal urinary and faecal incontinence and prolapse outcomes: randomised controlled trial. BJOG. 2014;121(1):112–20.
6. Byrd LM, Hobbiss JH, Tasker M. Is it possible to predict or prevent third degree tears? Color Dis. 2005;7(4):311–8.
7. Kettle C, Hills RK, Ismail KMK. Continuous versus interrupted sutures for repair of episiotomy or second degree tears. Cochrane Database Syst Rev. 2012;11:CD000947.
8. NICE. National Institute for Health and Clinical Excellence. Postnatal care: routine postnatal care for women and their babies. NICE Clinical Guideline No 37. 2006.
9. Bols EMJ, Hendriks EJM, Berghmans BCM, Baeten CGMI, Nijhuis JG, de Bie RA. A systematic review of etiological factors for postpartum fecal incontinence. Acta Obstet Gynecol Scand. 2010;89:302–14.
10. Klein MC, Gauthier RJ, Robbins JM, Kaczorowski J, Jorges SH, Franco ED, et al. Relationship of episiotomy to perineal trauma and morbidity, sexual dysfunction, and pelvic floor relaxation. Am J Obst Gynecol. 1994;171:591–8.
11. Al-Mufti R, McCarthy A, Fisk N. Survey of obstetricians' personal preference and discretionary practice. Eur J Obstet Gynecol Reprod Biol. 1997;73:1–4.
12. Dudley L, Kettle C, Ismail K. Prevalence, pathophysiology and current management of dehisced perineal wounds following childbirth. Br J Midwifery. 2013;21(3):160–71.
13. Perkins E, Tohill S, Kettle C, Bick D, Ismail K. Women's views of important outcomes following perineal repair. Proceedings of the International Conference of Obstetrics and Gynaecology, Montreal. 2008;115(Suppl 1):1.179 32.
14. Stock L, Basham E, Gossett D, Lewicky-Gaupp C. Factors associated with wound complications in women with obstetric anal sphincter injuries (OASIS). Am J Obstet Gynecol. 2013;208:327. e1–6
15. Lewicky-Gaupp C, Leader-Cramer A, Johnson LL, Kneton K. Wound complications after obstetric anal sphincter injuries. Obstet Gynaecol. 2015;125(5):1088–93.
16. Boyle M. Wound healing in midwifery. Oxford: Radcliffe; 2006.
17. Gray D, Cooper P. Nutrition and wound healing: what is the link? J Wound Care. 2001;10(3):86–9.
18. NICE. National Institute for Health and Clinical Excellence. Surgical site infection: prevention and treatment of surgical site infection clinical guideline 74. 2008.
19. Walburn JV, Vedhara K, Hankins M, Rixon L, Weinman J. Psychological stress and wound healing in humans: a systematic review and meta-analysis. J Psychosom Res. 2009;67(3):253–71.
20. Davidson N. REEDA:evaluation postpartum healing. J Nurse-Midwifery. 1974;XIX(2):196–8.
21. Alvarenga MB, Francisco AA, de Oliveira SMJV, da Silva FMB, Shimoda GT, Damiani LP. Episiotomy healing assessment: redness, oedema, ecchymosis, discharge, approximation (REEDA) scale reliability. Rev Lat-Am Enfermagem. 2015;23(1):162–8. doi:10.1590/0104-1169.3633.2538.
22. Patten H. Identifying wound infection: taking a wound swab. Wound Essentials. 2010;5:64–6.
23. Dudley L, Kettle C, Ismail K. Secondary suturing compared to non-suturing for broken down perineal wounds following childbirth. Cochrane Database Syst Rev. 2013;9:CD008977.
24. Dudley L, Kettle C, Carter P, Thomas P, Ismail KM. Perineal resuturing versus expectant management following vaginal delivery complicated by a dehisced wound (PREVIEW): protocol for a pilot and feasibility randomised controlled trial. BMJ Open. 2012;2(4):e001458.

25. CMACE. Centre for Maternal and Child Enquiries. Saving mothers' lives: reviewing maternal deaths to make motherhood safer; 2006–2008. The 8th report on confidential enquiries into maternal deaths in the UK. BJOG: Int J Obstet Gynaecol. 2011;118(Suppl 1):1–203.
26. Chandru S, Nafee T, Ismail K, Kettle C. Evaluation of modified Fenton procedure for persistent superficial dyspareunia following childbirth. Gynaecol Surg. 2010;7(3):245–8.
27. Mous M, Muller SA, De Leeuw JW. Long-term effects of anal sphincter rupture during vaginal delivery: faecal incontinence and sexual complaints. BJOG. 2008;115:234–8.
28. Rogers RG, Borders N, Leeman LM, Albers LL. Does spontaneous genital tract trauma impact postpartum sexual function? J Midwifery Women's Health. 2009;54(2):98–104.
29. Radestad I, Olsson A, Nissen E, Rubertsson C. Tears in the vagina, perineum, sphincter ani, and rectum and first sexual intercourse after childbirth: a nationwide follow-up. Birth. 2008;35(2):98–106.
30. Andrews V, Thacker R, Sultan A, Jones P. Evaluation of pospartum perineal pain and dyspareunia – a prospective study. Eur J Obstet Gynecol Reprod Biol. 2008;137:152–6.
31. Fodstad K, Laine K, Staff AC. Different episiotomy techniques, postpartum perineal pain, and blood loss: an observational study. Int Urogynecol J. 2013;24:865–72.
32. McDonald EA, Gartland D, Small R, Brown SJ. Dyspareunia and childbirth: a prospective cohort study. BJOG. 2015;122:672–9.
33. Fodstad K, Staff AC, Laine K. Sexual activity and dyspareunia the first year postpartum in relation to degree of perineal trauma. Int Urogynecol J. 2016;16 Epub ahead of print
34. Brummen H, Bruinse H, van de Pol G, Heintz A, van der Vaart C. Which factors determine the sexual function 1 year after childbirth? BJOG. 2006;113:914–8.
35. Olson A, Lundquist M, Faxelid E, Nissen E. Women's thoughts about sexual life after childbirth. Scand J Caring Sci. 2005;19:381–7.
36. Klein MC, Janssen PA, MacWilliam L, Kaczorowski J, Johnson B. Determinants of vaginal-perineal integrity and pelvic floor functioning in childbirth. Am J Obstet Gynecol. 1997;176(2):403–10.
37. Signorello LB, Harlow BL, Chekos AK, Repke JT. Postpartum sexual functioning and its relationship to perineal trauma: a retrospective cohort study of primiparous women. Am J Obstet Gynecol. 2001;184(5):881–90.
38. Andreucci CB, Bussadori JC, Pacagnella RC, Chou D, Filippi V, Say L, Cecatti JG, and on behalf of the Brazilian COMMAG Study Group and the WHO Maternal Morbidity Working Group. Sexual life and dysfunction after maternal morbidity: a systematic review. BMC Pregnancy Childbirth. 2015;15:307.
39. Stedenfeldt M, Pirhonen J, Blix E, Wilsgaard T, Vonen B, Øian P. Anal incontinence, urinary incontinence and sexual problems in primiparous women, a comparison between women with episiotomy only and women with episiotomy and obstetric anal sphincter injury. BMC Women's Health. 2014;14:157.
40. Gyhagen M, Bullarbo M, Nielsen TF, Milsom I. The prevalence of urinary incontinence 20 years after childbirth: a national cohort study in singleton primiparae after vaginal or caesarean delivery. BJOG. 2013;120(2):144–51.
41. Meyer S, Schreyer A, De Grandi P, Hohlfield P. The effects of birth on urinary continence mechanisms and other pelvic floor characteristics. Obstet Gynecol. 1998;92:613–8.
42. Toozs-Hobson P, Balmforth J, Cardozo L, Khullar V, Athanasiou S. The effect of mode of delivery on pelvic floor functional anatomy. Int Urogynecol J. 2008;19:407–16.
43. Meyer S, Bachelard O, De Gandi P. Do bladder neck mobility and urethral sphincter function differ during pregnancy compared with the non-pregnant state? Int Urogynecol J. 1998;9:397–404.
44. Mulder FE, Oude Rengerink K, van der Post JA, Hakvoort RA, Roovers JP. Delivery-related risk factors for covert postpartum urinary retention after vaginal delivery. Int Urogynecol J. 2016;27(1):55–60.
45. Mulder F, Schoffelmeer M, Hakvoort R, Limpens J, Mol B, van der Post J, Roovers J. Risk factors for postpartum urinary retention: a systematic review and meta-analysis. BJOG. 2012;119:1440–6.

46. Patel DA, Xiao X, Thomason AD, Ransom SB, Ivy JS, DeLancey JOL. Childbirth and pelvic floor dysfunction: an epidemiologic approach to the assessment of prevention opportunities at delivery. Am J Obstet Gynecol. 2006;195:23–8.
47. Rortveit G, Daltveit AK, Hannestad YS, Hunskaar S; for the Norwegian EPINCONT Study. Urinary incontinence after vaginal delivery or cesarean section. N Engl J Med. 2003;348:900–7.
48. Handa VL, Blomquist JL, McDermott KC, Friedman S, Muñoz A. Pelvic floor disorders after childbirth: effect of episiotomy, perineal laceration, and operative birth. Obstet Gynecol. 2012;119(2 Pt 1):233–9.
49. Andrews V, Shelmeridine S, Sultan AH, Thakar R. Anal and urinary incontinence 4 years after a vaginal delivery. Int Urogynecol J. 2013;24:55–60.
50. Working Party of the Royal College of Physicians. Incontinence. Causes, management and provision of services. London: J R Coll Phys; 1995.
51. Norton CCJ, Butler U, Harari D, Nelson RL, Pemberton J, et al. In: Ambrams PCL, Khoury S, Wein A, editors. Incontinence: second international consultation on incontinence. Plymouth: Health Publications Ltd; 2002. p. 987–1043.
52. Boreham M, Richter H, Kenton K, Nager C, Gregory W, Aronson M. Anal incontinence in women presenting for gynecologic care: prevalence, risk factors and impact upon quality of life. Am J Obstet Gynecol. 2005;192:1637–42.
53. Lo J, Osterweil P, Li H, Mori T, Eden K, Guise J. Quality of life in women with postpartum anal incontinence. Obstet Gynecol. 2010;115(4):809–14.
54. Leigh R, Turnberg L. Faecal incontinence: the unvoiced symptom. Lancet. 1982;1(8285):1349–51.
55. Sultan AH, Kamm MA, Hudson CN, Bartram CI. Third degree obstetric anal sphincter tears: risk factors and outcome of primary repair. BMJ. 1994;308(6933):887–91.
56. Nichols CM, Nam M, Ramakrishnan V, Lamb EH, Currie N. Anal sphincter defects and bowel symptoms in women with and without recognized anal sphincter trauma. Am J Obstet Gynecol. 2006;194(5):1450–5.
57. Fitzpatrick M, Behan M, O'Connell PR, O'Herlihy C. Randomised clinical trial to assess anal sphincter function following forceps or vacuum assisted vaginal delivery. BJOG: Int J Obstet Gynaecol. 2003;110(4):424–9.
58. MacArthur CBD, Keighley MR. Faecal incontinence after childbirth. BJOG. 1997;104:46–50.
59. Zetterstrom J, Lopez A, Anzen B, Dolk A, Norman M, Mellgren A. Anal incontinence after vaginal delivery; a prospective study in primiparous women. Br J Obstet Gynaecol. 1999;106(4):324–30.
60. Laine K, Skjeldestad FE, Sanda B, Horne H, Spydslaug A, Staff AC. Prevalence and risk factors for anal incontinence after obstetric anal sphincter rupture. Acta Obstet Gynecol Scand. 2011;90:319–24.
61. Visscher AP, Lam TJ, Hart N, Felt-Bersma RJF. Fecal incontinence, sexual complaints, and anorectal function after third-degree obstetric anal sphincter injury (OASI): 5-year follow-up. Int Urogynecol J. 2014;25:607–13.
62. Oude Lohuis EJ, Everhardt E. Outcome of obstetric anal sphincter injuries in terms of persisting endoanal ultrasonographic defects and defecatory symptoms. Int J Obstet Gynecol. 2014;126:70–3.
63. Reid AJ, Beggs AD, Sultan AH, Roos A-M, Thakar R. Outcome of repair of obstetric anal sphincter injuries after three years. Int J Obstet Gynecol. 2015;127:47–50.
64. Meyer I, Richter HE. Impact of fecal incontinence and its treatment on quality of life in women. Women's Health. 2015;11:225–38.
65. Koughnett V, Wexner SD. Current management of fecal incontinence: choosing amongst treatment options to optimize outcomes. World J Gastroenterol. 2013;19:9216–30.
66. Poskus T, Buzinsiene D, Drasutiene G, Samalavicius N, Barkus A, Barisauskiene A, et al. Haemorrhoids and anal fissures during pregnancy and after childbirth; a prospective cohort study. Br J Obstet Gynaecol. 2014;121:1666.

67. RCOG. Third- and fourth-degree perineal tears, management (Green-top 29). RCOG Greentop Guidelines. 2007;2:1.
68. Priddis H, Dahlen H, Schmied V. Women's experiences following severe perineal trauma: a meta-ethnographic synthesis. J Adv Nurs. 2013;69(4):748–60.
69. O'Reilly R, Peters K, Beale B, Jackson D. Women's experiences of recovery from childbirth: focus on pelvis problems that extend beyond the puerperium. J Clin Nurs. 2009;18:2013–9.
70. Williams A, Lavender T, Richmond DH, Tincello DG. Women's experiences after a third-degree obstetric anal sphincter tear: a qualitative study. Birth: Issues Perinatal Care. 2005;32(2):129–37.
71. Salmon D. A feminist analysis of women's experiences of perineal trauma in the immediate post-delivery period. Midwifery. 1999;15(4):247–56.
72. Grabowska C. Unhappiness after childbirth. In: Squire C, editor. The social context of birth. UK: Radcliffe Publishing; 2009. p. 236–50.
73. Priddis H, Schmied V, Dahlen H. Women's experiences following severe perineal trauma: a qualitative study. BMC Womens Health. 2014;14(1):32.
74. Way S. A qualititative study exploring women's personal experiences of their perineum after childbirth: expectations, reality and returning to normality. Midwifery. 2012;28(5):12–9.
75. East E, Sherburn M, Nagle C, Said J, Forster D. Perineal pain following childbirth: prevalence, effects on postnatal recovery and analgesia usage. Midwifery. 2012;28(1):93–8.
76. Rizk D, Hassan M, Shaheen J, Cherian J, Micallef R, Dunn E. The prevalence and determinants of health care-seeking behavior for fecal incontinence in multiparous United Arab Emirates females. Dis Colon Rectum. 2001;44:1850–6.
77. Woollett A, Nicolson P. Post-partum care and experiences of mothering. J Reprod Infant Psychol. 2007;15:85–9.

Chapter 9
Perineal Trauma and Pelvic Floor Muscle Training

Amallia Brair, Nina Bridges, and Khaled Ismail

Abstract There is a recognised association between pregnancy, in itself, and pelvic floor disorders. Currently there is high level evidence that structured antenatal pelvic floor muscle training reduces the risk of postnatal urinary incontinence. Studies have also reported on benefits of pelvic floor exercises in the physical recovery after childbirth particularly when commenced within the first month following higher grades of perineal trauma. However, most of this evidence relates to structured training programmes, which ensure that the woman is able to locate her pelvic floor muscles and that they are motivated and compliant. Referral to specialised obstetric physiotherapists tends to be reserved for symptomatic and high-risk women. Indeed, it would be unrealistic and not feasible for every pregnant woman to be seen by an obstetric physiotherapist. Therefore, with current demands on obstetricians and midwives, it is essential for maternity units to develop innovative care pathways to ensure the delivery of an effective prophylactic pelvic floor muscle training programme.

Keywords Pelvic floor exercises • Pelvic floor muscles • PFME • PFMT • physiotherapy

A. Brair • N. Bridges
Birmingham Women's NHS Foundation Trust, Birmingham, UK

K. Ismail (✉)
University of Birmingham, Birmingham, UK
e-mail: k.ismail@bham.ac.uk

K.M.K. Ismail (ed.), *Perineal Trauma at Childbirth*,
DOI 10.1007/978-3-319-14860-1_9

Introduction

There is a recognised association between pregnancy and pelvic floor disorders. Studies show that 25–30 % of women report urinary incontinence (UI) after childbirth. Moreover, the majority of women who have symptoms of incontinence by 3 months postnatal will continue to have this symptom and its negative impact on their quality of life in the longer term [1]. Data from the PErineal Assessment and Repair Longitudinal Study (PEARLS) involving 3,681 women showed that the reported incidence of UI in women following vaginal birth was 20 % and 25 % at 6 and 12 weeks postnatally respectively.

The pathogenesis of childbirth-related pelvic floor dysfunction is probably multifactorial, resulting from direct damage to the pelvic floor muscles, fascia and nerves during pregnancy and childbirth, which becomes increasingly problematic with increasing parity and age. A recent 12 year prospective cohort study demonstrated that after adjustment for parity, body mass index and age at first birth, women who delivered exclusively by caesarean section were less likely to have UI than those who only had spontaneous vaginal births; however, there was no significant difference between women who had all their births vaginally compared with those who had a combination of caesarean and spontaneous vaginal births [1]. Interestingly, even in the exclusive caesarean section group there were still as many as 40 % of women who reported symptoms of UI. Moreover, the authors of the above study reported that exclusive caesarean section confers no benefit for subsequent FI [1]. Therefore, this evidence highlights that the pregnancy itself is a risk factor for pelvic floor dysfunction. Hence deferring pelvic floor muscle training (PFMT) until the postnatal period misses out on a potentially important window of opportunity to sustain pelvic floor function.

Antenatal Pelvic Floor Muscle Training

Several mechanisms have been proposed with regard to mode of action of PFMT in preventing UI and pelvic floor dysfunction. It is believed that training muscles develops appropriate motor patterns and increases the muscle reserve which in turn reduces the likelihood of damage, its extent and even facilitates the recovery from any damage that ensues [2].

Based on the evidence above that a substantial proportion of women who were exclusively delivered by caesarean section have UI and FI symptoms it seems that pregnancy per se can have a negative impact on pelvic floor function [1]. It is postulated that antenatal PFMT can help to improve the function of the pelvic floor muscles and thus prevent UI and FI by counteracting the increased intra-abdominal pressure in pregnancy, the hormonally mediated reduction in urethral pressure and the increased laxity of fascia and ligaments in the pelvic area.

Several randomised controlled trials have evaluated the efficacy of PFMT as a preventive intervention in reducing the occurrence of UI secondary to pregnancy and childbirth [3–7]. A Cochrane review investigated the effectiveness of antenatal PFMT for prevention and treatment of urinary and faecal incontinence in pregnant and postnatal women [8]. The review included 22 trials involving 8,485 women and analysed the data according to whether PFMT interventions were for prevention of UI (pregnant women without prior UI), for treatment or were mixed prevention/treatment trials. The main findings were that, in prevention trials, pregnant women without prior UI who were randomised to PFMT and supervision were 30 % less likely than women randomised to no PFMT or usual antenatal care, to report UI up to 6 months after delivery. The effectiveness of the intervention in treatment and mixed trials was less clear. The review authors concluded it is possible that mixed prevention and treatment approaches might be effective when the intervention is intensive enough. Thus, currently the clearest evidence regarding PFMT and childbirth-related UI relates to the protective effect of routine antenatal PFMT in pregnant women without previous UI. Indeed the current recommendation in the UK is that all pregnant women should be provided with information about the exercises at their initial booking appointment.

There has been some concern amongst health care professionals about the impact of antenatal PFMT on labour and birth. This concern has stemmed from the anecdotal evidence that athletes who undertake regular strenuous physical exercise and women who undertake regular PFMT would have rigid and less elastic pelvic floor muscles which would contribute to prolongation of the second stage of labour and potentially higher risk of perineal trauma. However, when linking data collected from women participating in the Norwegian Mother and Child Birth Cohort Study to the Norwegian Birth Registry, Bø and colleagues concluded that pre-pregnancy and antenatal PFMT did not affect labour and birth outcomes or complication rates [9].

Moreover, a more recent study did not support the hypothesis that women exercising before and during pregnancy have a narrower levator hiatus (LH) area or more complicated childbirths than non-exercising women [10].

Postnatal PFMT

A study conducted in Norway tested the effect of postnatal exercises in strengthening the pelvic floor muscles (PFMs) and concluded that a specially devised PFMT programme can add significantly to physical recovery after childbirth [11]. Indeed, too much rest can be counterproductive, as muscles require a certain amount of movement to be able to recover in an efficient manner. Therefore as soon after birth as the woman is able to, she should be encouraged and supported to start PFM exercises, even if these are small contractions of muscles within their limit of pain. PFMT is expected to help in recovery in several ways. The repeated contractions and relaxations can cause a pumping action, which will lead to an increase in blood supply to the area hence facilitate healing. This pumping action will also help with venous and lymphatic drainage hence reducing the oedema and tension in the surrounding tissues. It is also suggested that PFM exercise can aid in reducing perineal pain through the Gate Control Theory of Pain (where a stimulus blocks the painful impulse from being conducted to the nervous system).

With regards to Obstetric Anal Sphincter Injuries (OASIS), early structured PFMT (within the first month postpartum) has been reported to offer additional benefits by reducing medium-term functional consequences of this complex trauma [12]. The authors of this chapter believe that such structured training should be delivered and supervised by specialised Obstetric/Women's Health physiotherapists to ensure the effectiveness of the training undertaken.

Assessing PFMT

Evaluation of PFM function is an essential component of any structured PFMT programme. Firstly, It ensures that the woman is able to locate and correctly perform a PFM contraction. Secondly, it enables the health care professional to give feedback and document any changes in PFM strength. There are several methods to objectively assess different aspects of pelvic floor function and strength:

1. Measures for the ability to locate and contract the PFMs:
    - Clinical observation of a perineal lift. If a woman cannot tolerate or refuses an internal examination then visible (by use of a mirror in case of a self assessment) or palpable perineal lift equates to pelvic floor activity.
    - Vaginal palpation by the woman after receiving instructions about self-examination or by the clinician. This is considered the routine assessment because it also enables evaluation of the strength of the contraction.
    - Coccygeal Movement Test (CMT). This is a potentially useful and less invasive test that relies on palpating the ventral movement of the coccyx with an accurate PFM contraction. This happens because of the posterior attachmenet of the medial fibres of the levator ani muscle to the coccyx (Pubo-coccygeous muscle) [13]. However, the diagnostic accuracy of this test remains under study.
    - Electromyography [EMG] using surface or internal electrodes to enable the woman to visualise the electrical activity of the muscles when contracting the PFMs.
    - Imaging the PFMs using ultrasound or MRI. Real – time ultrasound can also be used to measure the contraction with the probe placed either suprapubically, on the perineum or with the probe inserted into the vagina or rectum. Real- time MRI has also been used, however it is too expensive to be implemented as a routine measure.
2. Measures to quantify strength of muscle contraction: This could be achieved using a manual muscle test by vaginal palpation or by means of biofeedback using EMG or manometry, the latter is less commonly used now. The most accurate way of assessment is a digital vaginal examination of the pelvic floor

using a modified Oxford scale of strength 0–5 scale and the PERFECT scoring system- P= Power, E= Endurance, R= Repetitions, F= Fast twitch, ECT= Every Contraction Timed [14]. Pelvic floor muscle strength and endurance can be measured by measuring the squeeze pressure. Maximum strength can be measured by asking the patient to contract the pelvic floor muscles as hard as possible. Endurance can be measured by seeing for how long the patient can maintain the contraction or how many repetitive contractions can the patient do. The measurement can be done in the urethra, vagina, or rectum using manual muscle testing with vaginal palpation, pressure manometry, or dynamometry [15].

The Current Gap Between Evidence and Practice

In the UK the National Institute for Health and Clinical Excellence (NICE) antenatal care guidelines recommend that women are provided with information about pelvic floor exercises by their midwives during their initial booking appointment [16]. However, it is important to highlight that RCT evidence upon which this recommendation is based, relates to structured supervised PFMT programmes, some being fairly intensive. Therefore, one should be careful not to extrapolate this evidence to "providing information about pelvic floor exercises". This is of particular relevance because a significant number of women are not able to locate their pelvic floor muscles without supervised instruction. Indeed, a trial in Norway reported no benefit when PFMT were taught in a general fitness pregnancy class without individual instruction of correct PFMT contraction [17]. Moreover, pregnant women often report not recalling being given any advice to do PFMT and some of those who remember being informed about it could not remember that they were given instructions on how to do this and many of those who do get advice do not perform them [18]. Therefore, to be able to bridge the current gap between evidence and recommended practice it is imperative to address barriers and motivators of implementation of PFMT in day-to-day practice.

The Woman

The woman needs to be fully informed about the benefits of regular PFMT in maintaining and regaining pelvic floor muscle strength and muscle healing as well the potential short and long-term consequences of not doing so. The woman may also have some misinformation on how the exercises may negatively impact on birth and perineal trauma. This will ensure the woman has the required motivation to remember and undertake these exercises. Instructions about undertaking PFMT must be clear and delivered using different modalities to overcome any cultural, educational, social, financial or language barriers.

The Organisation and Health Care Professionals

Maternity healthcare professionals have an essential role to ensure the delivery of an effective PFMT programme. However, with the ever increasing demands on maternity staff to deliver other aspects of care to mothers and babies, this can sometimes be challenging. It will be unrealistic to expect that every pregnant woman would see a specialised obstetric physiotherapist during the course of her pregnancy to ensure that women are provided with expert guidance with regards to PFMT. Indeed with the current levels of service demands on physiotherapists it is more effective to utilise their expertise for the cohort of women who are symptomatic, suffered complex perineal trauma or those who are at high risk of pelvic floor dysfunction. Therefore, it is important for individual maternity units to consider realistic, effective and efficient ways to deliver such service.

Conclusion

Evidence for the benefit of antenatal and postnatal PFMT in reducing childbirth-related pelvic floor dysfunction exists. However, this evidence relates to structured training programmes which involve clear instructions, an objective measure of ability to locate the PFMs and regular visits to ensure compliance. It is important to consider innovative ways of addressing the current gap between evidence and practice to ensure its effective implementation.

References

1. MacArthur C, Glazener C, Lancashire R, Herbison P, Wilson D. Exclusive caesarean section delivery and subsequent urinary and faecal incontinence: a 12-year longitudinal study. BJOG: Int J Obstet Gynaecol. 2011;118(8):1001–7. Epub 2011/04/12.
2. Hay-Smith J, Morkved S, Fairbrother KA, Herbison GP. Pelvic floor muscle training for prevention and treatment of urinary and faecal incontinence in antenatal and postnatal women. Cochrane Database Syst Rev. 2008;4:CD007471. Epub 2008/10/10.
3. Gorbea Chavez V, Velázquez Sánchez Mdel P, Kunhardt Rasch JR. Effect of pelvic floor exercise during pregnancy and puerperium on prevention of urinary stress incontinence [Efecto de los ejercicios del piso pelvico durante el embarazoy el puerperio en la prevencion de la incontinencia urinaria de esfuerzo]. Ginecol Obstet Mex. 2004;72(12):628–36.
4. Sampselle CM, Miller JM, Mims BL, Delancey JO, Ashton-Miller JA, Antonakos CL. Effect of pelvic muscle exercise on transient incontinence during pregnancy and after birth. Obstet Gynecol. 1998;91(3):406–12. Epub 1998/03/10.
5. Morkved S, Bo K, Schei B, Salvesen KA. Pelvic floor muscle training during pregnancy to prevent urinary incontinence: a single-blind randomized controlled trial. Obstet Gynecol. 2003;101(2):313–9. Epub 2003/02/11.
6. Stothers L. A randomized trial to evaluate effectiveness and cost effectiveness of naturopathic cranberry products as prophylaxis against urinary tract infection in women. Can J Urol. 2002;9(3):1558–62. Epub 2002/07/18.

7. Reilly ET, Freeman RM, Waterfield MR, Waterfield AE, Steggles P, Pedlar F. Prevention of postpartum stress incontinence in primigravidae with increased bladder neck mobility: a randomised controlled trial of antenatal pelvic floor exercises. BJOG Int J Obstet Gynaecol. 2002;109(1):68–76. Epub 2002/02/16.
8. Boyle R, Hay-Smith EJC, Cody JD, Mørkved S. Pelvic floor muscle training for prevention and treatment of urinary and faecal incontinence in antenatal and postnatal women. Cochrane Database of Systematic Reviews 2012, Issue 10. Art. No.: CD007471. DOI: 10.1002/14651858. CD007471.pub2.
9. Bo K, Fleten C, Nystad W. Effect of antenatal pelvic floor muscle training on labor and birth. Obstet Gynecol. 2009;113:1279–84.
10. Bø K, Hilde G, Stær-Jensen J, Siafarikas F, Tennfjord MK, Engh ME. Does general exercise training before and during pregnancy influence the pelvic floor "opening" and delivery outcome? A 3D/4D ultrasound study following nulliparous pregnant women from mid-pregnancy to childbirth. Br J Sports Med. 2015;49:196–9.
11. Mørkved S, Bø K. The effect of post-natal exercises to strengthen the pelvic floor muscles. Acta Obstet Gynecol Scand. 1996;75(4):382–5. PMID:8638461.
12. Mathe M, Valancogne G, Atallah A, Sciard C, Doret M, Gaucherand P, Beaufils E. Early pelvic floor muscle training after obstetrical anal sphincter injuries for the reduction of anal incontinence. Eur J Obstet Gynecol Reprod Biol. 2016;199:201–6.
13. Stensgaard SH, Moeller Bek K, Ismail KM. Coccygeal movement test: an objective, noninvasive test for localization of the pelvic floor muscles in healthy women. Med Princ Pract. 2014;23(4):318–22. doi:10.1159/000362337. Epub 2014 May 15. PMID: 24852386.
14. Laycock J, Jerwood D. Pelvic floor muscle assessment: the PERFECT scheme. Physiotherapy. 2001;87(12):631–42.
15. Bø K, Sherburn M. Evaluation of female pelvic-floor muscle function and strength. Physical Therapy. 2005;85(3):269–82.
16. National Institute of Health and Care Excellence. Antenatal Care Guideline (CG62). 2008. http://www.nice.org.uk/guidance/cg62.
17. Bo K, Haakstad LEH. Is pelvic muscle training effective when taught in a general fitness class in pregnancy? A randomised controlled trial. Physiotherapy. 2011;97:190–5.
18. MacArthur C, Ismail K. Commentary on 'prevention of postpartum stress incontinence in primigravidae with increased bladder neck mobility: a randomised controlled trial of antenatal pelvic floor exercises'. BJOG. 2014;121(Suppl 7):67–72. doi:10.1111/1471-0528.13150. PMID: 25488091.

Chapter 10
Management of Perineal Trauma Complications: The Role of the MDT

Kaori Futaba, Simon Radley, Sara Webb, and Matthew Parsons

Abstract The functionality of the Pelvic floor is a result of its complex anatomical structure and integrated physiological mechanisms. Women who sustain OASIS may have co-existing problems or develop new symptoms that require the involvement of many specialists, such as urogynaecologists, colorectal surgeons, physiotherapists, gastrologists, radiographers. The aim of this chapter is to provide an outline of how Multi-Disciplinary Team (MDT) working is best placed, not only to provide women with pelvic floor disorders timely access to necessary investigations, services and management options, but also to develop specialism in related professions, such as midwifery, for the improvement in patient centred care. It provides examples of MDT models of case review meetings and combined MDT outpatient clinics that could be replicated in different units of all caseload sizes.

Keywords Pelvic floor • Multidisciplinary team • Combined clinic • Perineal trauma • OASIS

K. Futaba (✉) • S. Radley
Department of Surgery, University Hospital Birmingham, Mindelsohn Way, Edgbaston, Birmingham B15 2WB, UK
e-mail: kaori.futaba@uhb.nhs.uk; simon.radley@uhb.nhs.uk

S. Webb
Birmingham Women's NHS Foundation Trust, Edgbaston, Birmingham B15 2TG, UK
e-mail: sara.webb@bwnft.nhs.uk

M. Parsons
Department of Urogynaecology, Birmingham Women's NHS Foundation Trust, Edgbaston, Birmingham B15 2TG, UK
e-mail: matthew.parsons@bwnft.nhs.uk

K.M.K. Ismail (ed.), *Perineal Trauma at Childbirth*,
DOI 10.1007/978-3-319-14860-1_10

Introduction

Pelvic floor pathology in women encompasses a wide spectrum of functional, anatomical, neurological, hormonal and neoplastic conditions which may be associated with symptoms of bowel, urinary and/or sexual dysfunction [1]. The realisation that the pelvic floor does not exist in isolation is an important concept which must be explored [2]. Traditionally, the pelvis has been anatomically and functionally divided into three 'compartments', namely, an anterior (the bladder), a middle (the vagina) and a posterior (the rectum), with each compartment being cared for in isolation. However, what has become increasingly apparent and suggested for over two decades is that pelvic floor disorders would be better managed through the collaborative efforts of obstetricians, gynaecologists, midwives, urologists, colorectal surgeons, psychologists, physiotherapists, neurologists, and radiologists [3]. Women who sustain an anal sphincter injury may well have co-existent or develop future symptoms in other compartments and as such, a Multidisciplinary Team (MDT) approach is best placed to coordinate their care. Research has been published expressing the need for a dedicated multi-disciplinary clinic for review of all women who sustain Obstetric Anal Sphincter Injuries (OASIS) in the postnatal period [4–6]. This chapter will discuss the role of the MDT in the management of OASIS and childbirth related Pelvic Floor disorders, giving examples of how it can work in practice and the Role of the Specialist Perineal Midwife in management of women with OASIS.

The Role of the MDT for Women with OASIS

There are many benefits in developing a MDT approach for follow up of anal sphincter injuries. The Calman-Hine report, 1995, proposed a MDT approach for the management of colorectal cancer which is now well established [7], and MDT working already plays a key role in the management of benign diseases such as inflammatory bowel disease.

The members of a Pelvic Floor/OASIS MDT need to be inclusive and represent the many specialisms needed (Box 10.1) [8–10]. This facilitates the necessary open multi-disciplinary discussion necessary to benefit women with more complex problems, particularly when more than one pelvic compartment is affected. The team can share ideas and experiences to reach a consensus on the best treatment options, some of which may involve joint surgical procedures. It is estimated that one in nine women will undergo surgery for pelvic floor disorders during their lifetime and that 30 % of these patients will require further surgery for the same condition [11]. With pelvic floor disorders, the correlation between structural abnormality and function is not always straightforward [12]. Organ specific approach in the management of pelvic floor disorders may result in partial treatment of their global pelvic floor dysfunction leading to high recurrence rate [8]. As Harold Drutz, ex-president of the

International Urogynaecological Association, at the 21st annual clinical meeting in Vienna, 1996, commented "we have done women a tremendous disservice by fractionating health care for pelvic floor disorders and there needs to be increasing dialogue, not monologue, between urologists, urogynaecologist, gynaecologists and colorectal surgeons" [13].

An interdisciplinary, multi-professional Pelvic Floor/OASIS Team, through regular case review meetings and combined out-patient clinics, provides an excellent environment for the development of collective expertise, facilitates evidence-led practice and improves patient care and satisfaction [9]. It provides a valuable way of managing difficult cases as well as streamlining treatment [11].

Box 10.1 Members of a Pelvic Floor/OASIS MDT

Urogynaecologists

- To offer specialist input into the investigation and management of conditions affecting the anterior and middle compartment.

Colorectal Surgeons *with specialist interest in pelvic floor disorders*

- To offer specialist input into the investigation and management of conditions affecting the posterior compartment.

Urologists *with specialist interest in pelvic floor disorders*

- To offer specialist input into the investigation and management of conditions affecting the anterior compartment.

Specialist Radiologists and radiographers

- Expert interpretation of specialised investigations such as transit study, defecating proctogram and MR proctogram.

Medical Gastroenterologists *with interest in dysmotility.*

- Gastroenterologists play a key role in the medical management of patients with functional bowel disorders. Most male and nulliparous women present through the medical clinic.

Physiologist

- Carries out GI physiology investigations including endorectal ultrasound scans and anorectal physiology. They may also be involved in programming and follow up of patients with sacral nerve stimulators.

Midwives *with specialist expertise in managing patients who have sustained previous obstetric sphincter injuries*

– Play an important role in supporting patients at a challenging time post obstetric injuries but also in counseling patients who has had previous obstetric injury decide how to deliver with subsequent pregnancies.

Specialist Nurses *with interest in managing pelvic floor dysfunction such as urinary or faecal incontinence.*

– Play a key role in providing patients support, education and teaching patients how to perform some of the conservative treatments such as self-catheterising and rectal irrigations. Helps to reinforce the advice given by the rest of the MDT in clinics.

Physiotherapists

– Offers postpartum pelvic floor rehabilitation, as well as targeted biofeedback sessions for patients with incontinence.

Dieticians

– Offers patients advice on dietary intake, which may have a profound effect on their abdominal and bowel symptoms.

Clinical Psychologists

– Some patients may have complex psychological issues, who would benefit from combined treatment with psychologists. Behavioural modification techniques are just as important as surgical treatments [10].

Chronic Pain specialists

– Patients with chronic pain, not managed by simple measures may benefit from assessment and other alternative treatments by the chronic pain team.

Examples of Models of Running a Pelvic Floor/OASIS MDT

MDT Case Review Meetings

MDT case review meetings provide a forum to discuss individual patients to ensure that the right treatment/management option is being offered to the patient. For complex patients in whom a surgical solution for their symptoms may not be possible, the knowledge that their cases have been discussed with all members of the MDT may help them accept proffered treatment suggestions more readily. It also allows standardisation of care across different units, building a link between different specialties and simplifying referral pathways. It is important to remember that the Pelvic Floor/OASIS MDT is not just about 'meeting' but is integral to providing the appropriate patient-centred care. In the authors' unit, case review meetings takes place on a monthly basis with sufficient time set aside to discuss the cases properly. On line patient records and radiological imaging allow us to discuss patients and their imaging and investigations. Careful notes from each member of the team are kept and letters detailing discussion and decisions are written to the patients' primary care physician, other involved parties and copied to the patient.

MDT 'Combined' Outpatient Clinics

A 'combined' MDT clinic allows key specialisms to be present in one clinic and consequently offer several advantages for both patients and clinicians. They enable the clinician in charge of the patient's dominant symptom to coordinate assessment and treatment, provide adequate time for comprehensive clinical assessment with immediate review and discussion of results to decide on best treatment plan, moreover, patients need only attend one out-patient clinic. Identifying symptomatic women in the combined clinic allows them early access to investigation and treatments (most of which are non-surgical) as well as appropriate support and counseling as required. Adjacency of clinic rooms means that advice is readily available from the subspecialists present as required. Combined clinics also offer a comprehensive training opportunity for junior staff and students.

Whilst the benefits of a combined clinic may seem evident, such clinics are labour intensive to run and manage. They are also perceived, at least initially, as not cost effective in overall healthcare delivery, especially for smaller healthcare providers. However, the joint clinic enables patients to be managed efficiently between specialisms, thus avoiding multiple trips to different hospitals for investigations, clinic appointments and the inconvenience and time delay resulting in waiting several weeks in between each appointment episode. A telephone survey performed on 165 patients' experience with the multidisciplinary pelvic floor clinic in Canada showed that the majority of patients were satisfied and accepting of a multidisciplinary approach to pelvic floor dysfunction [14]. Consequently, combined MDT clinics are cost effective and provide improved patient satisfaction in the long term, overall healthcare setting. In our unit, patients who have sustained OASIS are routinely reviewed 12 weeks postpartum in the dedicated MDT Obstetric Anal Sphincter Injury Services (OASIS) clinic. Consultants Obstetricians, Urogynaecologists, Colorectal Surgeons, Specialist incontinence Nurse and a Specialist Perineal Midwife, all members of the MDT OASIS/Pelvic Floor Team, staff this clinic [15]. To enable all specialisms to regularly attend, the clinic runs once a month.

Lower urinary tract symptoms and minor anal (other than incontinence) or vaginal symptoms are particularly common in this group of women. However, a review performed by Davis and Kumar in 2003 found that patients only reported their most severe symptoms and often did not report symptoms of incontinence or sexual

Delivery

Patients age at devivery
Date of delivery causing OASI
Hospital delivered at
Baby weight (in kgs)

Delivery: NVD Kiwi Forceps (*state type*):

Type of repair: Sphincter not repaired End-to-end Overlap Not specified
3A 3B 3C 4C Unspecified

Bowel Symptoms

Frequency of opening bowels: .... per day or .... per week
Consistency of motion: watery sloppy soft and formed hard
Time can defer: .... minutes
Warning: Always Sometimes Never
Blood: On wiping PR/On stool: Frequently Sometimes Never
Mucus: On wiping PR/On stool: Frequently Sometimes Never
Urgency: Frequently Sometimes Never
Incontinence: Yes No
Consistency of incontinence: Solid Liquid Mucus
Passiive incontinence: Yes No
Nocturnal incontinence: Yes No
Control of flatus: Good Variable Poor
Incomplete evacuation: Always Sometimes Never
Pain: On defaecation Abdominally

Urinary Symptoms

Stress incontinence: Yes No
Urgency: Yes No
Frequency: ¼ ¼ 1 2 3 4 5 hrly
Nocturia: Yes .... times per night No

Sexual Function

Resumed Intercourse: Yes No
Dyspareunia: Yes No
Contraception: Yes (state method:) No

Breast Feeding Yes No

Examination: Accepted Declined Not performed

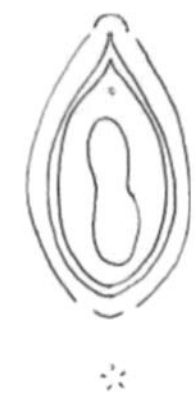

Anal Fissures seen: Yes No

Plan of care:

Anorectal manometry/USS Yes Declined
Physio referral Yes Declined
Follow up in OASIS Clinic in *or* Discharged
Treatment/medication:

Signed: Grade: Date:

Fig. 10.1 Patient history sheet – OASIS combined clinic

dysfunction as they felt it was not worthy of attention [16]. Therefore, at their initial appointment, all women are seen by a MDT clinician who completes a clinic specific patient history sheet (Fig. 10.1) that encompasses all pelvic floor compartments and helps identify any problems. It is fundamental to remember that the history sheet is there as a 'guide' for the consultation to ensure all relevant information is elicited. There is a risk that clinicians not familiar with such a sheet may interpret it as a 'tick box' exercise and feel they have used it appropriately simply asking the questions rather than interpreting and actioning the answers [17]. The history sheet also acts as a useful patient management audit tool to ensure treatment standards and compliance.

As well as the history sheet, patients are asked to complete a validated questionnaire to assess the severity score of bowel and urinary symptoms and its impact on Quality of Life (QoL) (Table 10.1). This is extremely important as what may be viewed as 'bothersome' by a clinician can be regarded as completely acceptable and normal to the patient, and vice versa [18]. This questionnaire can then be completed again throughout stages of treatment to assess progress.

Following discussion all women are offered further investigations (endoanal ultrasound and anal manometry) and physiotherapy assessment. Most will not require any interventions other than advice and reassurance and can be discharged from the clinic. However, women with ongoing concerns are kept under the care of the combined clinic or referred to a single specialist if appropriate.

Table 10.1 **(a–c)** Quality of life questionnaires

Recommended questionnaires for UI and UI/LUTS/OAB in women [18]		
Combined symptoms and QOL impact of UI	**Combined symptoms and QOL of OAB**	**QOL impact of UI**
BFLUTS-SF [20]	OAB-q [21] (grade Anew)	I-QOL [22, 23]
SUIQQ [24] (grade Anew)	UDI [25]	KHQ [26]
ICIQ [27]	UDI-6 [28]	IIQ [29]
	Incontinence Severity Index [30]	IIQ-7 [28]
	BFLUTS [31]	
Recommended questionnaires for symptoms and QOL impact of anal incontinence in women [18]		
Grade A	**Grade B**	**Grade C**
None	Faecal Incontinence Quality of Life scale (FIQL) [32]	Wexner incontinence grading scale [33]
	Manchester health questionnaire (MHQ) [34]	St Marks incontinence scores [35]
	Birmingham bowel and urinary symptoms questionnaire [1]	
Recommended questionnaires for symptoms and QOL impact of vaginal and pelvic floor problems [18]		
Grade A	**Grade B**	**Grade C**
None	PF distress inventory [36]	P-QOL/St. Mary's questionnaire [37]
	PF impact questionnaire [36]	PF dysfunction questionnaire [38]
		Electronic PF symptoms assessment questionnaire (e-PAQ) [39]
		ICIQ-VS [40]

The Development of the Specialist Perineal Midwife Role

One of the authors undertook to start and develop the role of Specialist Perineal Midwife in 2004 in order to form part of our hospital's MDT OASIS clinic. The expertise required for this role was facilitated and supported by consultants in obstetrics, gynaecology, and colo-rectal surgery, for the benefit of women, midwives and medical staff. The aim was to build a department that is not only centred on the needs of women but to expand the facility to provide services previously unavailable.

The OASIS Discussion Clinic was the initial development of the role and was set up to discuss and formalise a 'mode of delivery' plan for women with previous OASIS [19]. As well as providing women with the opportunity to discuss their previous delivery and agree on a mode of delivery for their subsequent pregnancy, the clinic has also enabled us to capture previously unavailable, but much needed data, in this area as research into this area is very limited.

Women's ability to make sensible and informed decisions about mode of subsequent delivery is certainly reflected in our data with a vaginal delivery rate of 60 % and an elective caesarean section rate of 40 % for women with previous OASI. Interestingly, during an enforced absence for illness, counseling was undertaken for a period of time by different members of the medical staff and the elective caesarean section rate increased to 53 %. This was despite a slight decrease in the number of symptomatic women for whom caesarean section was the most suitable choice. This highlights not just the importance of specialised knowledge for assisting women to make the most appropriate decision but also how this knowledge, and its use in communicating information and having discussions with women about the options, takes time to develop. Consequently the need for the Specialist Perineal Midwife to be involved in training and service delivery has been acknowledged and is ongoing.

A secondment with the Urogynaecology department has provided the skills and knowledge necessary for the specialist midwife role to encompass women with pregnancy related pelvic floor problems. This helps women who present with urine retention, continence issues or who need to be taught how to perform intermittent self catheterisation. As with OASIS, the numbers of women who present with these conditions might be perceived as relatively small but the emphasis for care provision must take into account the impact of the symptoms on the quality of their life. This can be considerable and it is essential to provide specialist skills in order to give the support that is needed.

The Specialist Perineal Midwife: Role Summary

- Postnatal MDT OASIS Clinic
- Antenatal OASIS Discussion Clinic
- Producing OASIS and postnatal perineal care information leaflets for women
- Link for midwives and medical staff requiring information and support
- Developing and teaching Perineal Suturing workshops
- Reviewing women with pregnancy related pelvic floor related problems
- Expanding the OASIS service to women to include midwife-led anal ultrasounds
- Promoting work at national and international conferences
- Research into long term symptoms from OASIS and BASIS (Birth After Sphincter Injuries)

Conclusion

The delivery of a modern pelvic floor service is more demanding and complex than ever. An effective service requires a group of enthusiastic clinicians and allied healthcare professionals with an interest in managing patients with pelvic floor disorder to work in tandem. We believe that for women with OASIS/Pelvic floor problems there is a role for a combined clinic but, as a minimum the use of the regular MDT meeting and global symptoms scoring systems allows identification of patients who will derive most benefit from multidisciplinary management. The unit also requires the basic diagnostic infrastructure and provision of a comprehensive range of treatments. Patients can be diagnosed accurately and treatment options can then be discussed with adequate information on realistic outcomes and possible complications. The spectrum of therapeutic options in pelvic floor conditions has increased enormously in the last decade, offering an exciting challenge for the future [9].

References

1. Hiller L, Radley S, Mann CH, Radley SC, Begum G, Pretlove SJ, et al. Development and validation of a questionnaire for the assessment of bowel and lower urinary tract symptoms in women. BJOG Int J Obstet Gynaecol. 2002;109(4):413–23.
2. Williams NS. Pelvic floor disorders and reconstruction – what next? Dis Colon Rectum. 2008;51(9):1309–11.
3. Wall LL, DeLancey JO. The politics of prolapse: a revisionist approach to disorders of the pelvic floor in women. Perspect Biol Med. 1991;34(4):486–96.
4. Fowler G, Williams A, Murphy G, Taylor K, Wood C, Adams E. How to set up a perineal clinic. Obstet Gynaecol. 2009;11:129–32.
5. Fernando RJ, Williams AA, Adams EJ. RCOG green top guidelines: management of third and fourth degree perineal tears following vaginal delivery. 2007. www.rcog.org.uk/guidelines.
6. Pretlove S, Thompson PJ, Toozs-Hobson R, Radley S. The first 18 months of a new perineal trauma clinic. J Obstet Gynaecol. 1997;24:399–402.
7. Calman KH, Hine D. Chief Medical Officers' Expert Advisory Group on Cancers: A policy framework for commissioning cancer services. London: Department of Health and Welsh Office. 1995.
8. Mirnezami A, Pilkington S, Monga A, Nugent KP. Multidisciplinary team meetings for pelvic floor disorders. Colorectal Dis Off J Assoc Coloproctol Great Brit Irel. 2008;10(4):413.
9. IN L, K N, Dixon T, editors. Pelvic floor disorders for the colorectal surgeon. Oxford: Oxford University Press; 2011.
10. Strohbehn K. Urogynecology. Curr Opin Obstet Gynecol. 1997;9(5):307–8.
11. Kenton K, Mueller ER. The global burden of female pelvic floor disorders. BJU Int. 2006;98(Suppl 1):1–5. ; discussion 6–7
12. Chatoor D, Soligo M, Emmanuel A. Organising a clinical service for patients with pelvic floor disorders. Best Pract Res Clin Gastroenterol. 2009;23(4):611–20.
13. Drutz HP. The first century of urogynecology and reconstructive pelvic surgery: where do we go from here? Presidential address, 21st annual Clinical Meeting, International Urogynecological Association, Vienna, Austria, 2–5 September 1996. Int Urogynecol J Pelvic Floor Dysfunct. 1996;7(6):348–53.
14. Chan MC, Schulz JA, Flood CG, Rosychuk RJ. A retrospective review of patients seen in a multidisciplinary pelvic floor clinic. J Obstet Gynaecol Can JOGC =J d'obstetrique et gynecologie du Canada JOGC. 2010;32(1):35–40.
15. Pretlove S, Thompson PJ, Toozs-Hobson PM, Radley S. The first 18 months of a new perineal trauma clinic. J Obstet Gynaecol: J Inst Obstet Gynaecol. 2004;24(4):399–402.
16. Davis K, Kumar D. Pelvic floor dysfunction: a conceptual framework for collaborative patient-centred care. J Adv Nurs. 2003;43(6):555–68.

17. Webb S, Futaba K, Burton C, Radley S, Parsons M, Toozs-Hobson P. Color Dis. 2012;14(33):1462–8910.
18. Avery KNL, Bosch JLHR, Gotoh M, Naughton M, Jackson S, Radley SC, Valiquette L, Batista J, Donovan J. Questionnaires to assess urinary and anal incontinence: review and recommendations. J Urol. 2007;177:39–49.
19. Webb S, Parsons M, Toozs-Hobson P. The role of specialised birth plans for women with previous third or fourth obstetric anal sphincter injuries (OASIS). MIDIRS. 2007;17(3):353–4.
20. Brookes ST, Donovan JL, Wright M, Jackson S, Abrams P. A scored form of the Bristol female lower urinary tract symptoms questionnaire: data from a randomized controlled trial of surgery for women with stress incontinence. Am J Obstet Gynecol. 2004;191:73.
21. Coyne K, Revicki D, Hunt R, Corey R, Stewart W, Bentkover J, et al. Psychometric validation of an overactive bladder symptom and health-related quality of life questionnaire: the OAB-q. Qual Life Res. 2002;11:563.
22. Wagner TH, Patrick DL, Bavendam TG, Martin ML, Buesching DP. Quality of life of persons with urinary incontinence: development of a new measure. Urology. 1996;47:67.
23. Patrick DL, Martin ML, Bushnell DM, Yalcin I, Wagner TH, Buesching DP. Quality of life of women with urinary incontinence: further development of the incontinence quality of life instrument (I-QOL). Urology. 1999;53:71.
24. Kulseng-Hanssen S, Borstad E. The development of a questionnaire to measure the severity of symptoms and the quality of life before and after surgery for stress incontinence. BJOG. 2003;110:983.
25. Shumaker SA, Wyman JF, Uebersax JS, McClish D, Fantl JA. Health-related quality of life measures for women with urinary incontinence: the incontinence impact questionnaire and the urogenital distress inventory. Qual Life Res. 1994;3:291.
26. Kelleher CJ, Cardozo LD, Khullar V, Salvatore S. A new questionnaire to assess the quality of life of urinary incontinent women. BJOG. 1997;104:1374.
27. Avery K, Donovan J, Peters T, Shaw C, Gotoh M, Abrams P. ICIQ: a brief and robust measure for evaluating the symptoms and impact of urinary incontinence. Neurourol Urodyn. 2004;23:322.
28. Uebersax JS, Wyman JF, Shumaker SA, McClish DK, Fantl AJ. Short forms to assess life quality and symptom distress for urinary incontinence in women: the incontinence impact questionnaire and the urogenital distress inventory. Continence program for women research group. Neurourol Urodyn. 1995;14:131.
29. Mouritsen L, Larsen JP. Symptoms, bother and POPQ in women referred with pelivic organ prolapse. Int Urogynecol J Pelvic Floor Dysfunct. 2004;14:122.
30. Sandvik H, Hunskaar S, Seim A, Hermstad R, Vanvik A, Bratt H. Validation of a severity index in female urinary incontinence and its implementation in an epidemiological survey. J Epidemiol Community Health. 1993;47:497.
31. Jackson S, Donovan J, Brookes S, Eckford S, Swithinbank L, Abrams P. The Bristol female lower urinary tract symptoms questionnaire: development and psychometric testing. Br J Urol. 1996;77:805.
32. Rockwood TH, Church JM, Fleshman JW, Kane RL, Mavrantonis C, Thorson AG, et al. Patient and surgeon ranking of the severity of symptoms associated with fecal incontinence: the fecal incontinence severity index. Dis Colon Rectum. 1999;42(12):1525–32.
33. Jorge JM, Wexner SD. Etiology and management of fecal incontinence. Dis Colon Rectum. 1993;36(1):77–97.
34. Bugg GJ, Kiff ES, Hosker G. A new condition-specific health-related quality of life questionnaire for the assessment of women with anal incontinence. BJOG. 2001;108:1057.
35. Vaizey CJ, Carapeti E, Cahill JA, Kamm MA. Prospective comparison of faecal incontinence grading systems. Gut. 1999;44(1):77–80.
36. Barber MD, Kuchibhatla MN, Pieper CF, Bump RC. Psychometric evaluation of 2 comprehensive condition-specific quality of life instruments for women with pelvic floor disorders. Am J Obstet Gynecol. 2001;185:1388.

37. Digesu GA, Santamato S, Khullar V, Santillo V, Digesu A, Cormio G, et al. Validation of an Italian version of the prolapse quality of life questionnaire. Eur J Obstet Gynecol Reprod Biol. 2003;106:184.
38. Ellerkmann R, Cundiff G, Melick C, Nihira M, Leffler K, Bent A. Correlation of symptoms with location and severity of pelvic organ prolapse. Am J Obstet Gynecol. 2001;185:1332.
39. Radley SC, Jones GL, Tanguy EA, Stevens VG, Nelson C, Mathers NJ. Computer interviewing in urogynaecology: concept, development and psychometric testing of an electronic pelvic floor assessment questionnaire in primary and secondary care. BJOG. 2006;113:231.
40. Price N, Jackson SR, Avery K, Brookes ST, Abrams P. Development and psychometric evaluation of the ICIQ waginal symptoms questionnaire: the ICIQ-VS. BJOG Int J Obstet Gynaecol. 2006;113(6):700–12.

Chapter 11
Role of Training to Reduce Perineal Trauma at an Organsiational Level

Katariina Laine and Sari Räisänen

Abstract In this chapter a process of changing clinical practice is presented with help of change management theory. The chapter is based on experiences from Norwegian hospitals in implementing a change in clinical practice during second stage of labour to reduce the incidence of obstetric anal sphincter injuries (OASIS). Training and educating Norwegian midwives and doctors on the labour wards to protect perineum during second stage of labour achieved the reduced incidence of OASIS. The educational programme included the entire staff involved in intra-partum care, both doctors and midwives, regardless of their length of experience in maternity practice. It is well recognised that educational programmes aiming to change an existing practice to a new method is a challenging process, hence, enthusiasm, leadership and resources are paramount.

Keywords Education • Change management • Manual perineal protection • Implementation

Introduction

To be able to offer the best practice with lowest possible complication rates and to improve health care quality, health care organisations, such as maternity units and birth centres, should continuously monitor the quality of care they deliver by

K. Laine (✉)
Department of Obstetrics, Oslo University Hospital, Ullevål, Norway
e-mail: kattiksen@yahoo.no

S. Räisänen
University of Helsinki, Helsinki, Finland
e-mail: shraisanen@gmail.com

K.M.K. Ismail (ed.), *Perineal Trauma at Childbirth*,
DOI 10.1007/978-3-319-14860-1_11

comparing their outcomes to recognised quality indicators. In the Organisation for Economic Co-operation and Development (OECD) countries, frequency of obstetric anal sphincter injuries (OASIS) is one such quality indicator [1]. Several hospitals in Norway have published results of reduced incidence of OASIS after implementing a change in management of the second stage of labour by training the staff to enhanced techniques to be adopted at birth [2–5]. The main change in these hospitals has been a change in clinical practice during the last part of second stage of labour. The implemented package of care consists of education and training in improved bimanual hands-on technique for manual perineal protection (MPP) together with better communication with the mother and using mediolateral or lateral episiotomy by indication only.

Such a change in clinical practice during delivery has become common in most Norwegian hospitals and this change was associated with a notable reduction in the national OASIS rate from 4.1 % in 2004 to 2.3 % in 2010 [6], and further to 1.7 % in 2015 [7]. Nevertheless, there are still some discrepancy in observed OASIS rates among different Norwegian maternity units [6, 7]. More recently, the Norwegian training programme has been adopted within units in other countries. Indeed, results from single hospitals in Denmark [8] and the UK [9] have already been published.

In this chapter, we describe the steps we have undertaken to change practice during second stage of labour among maternity staff in a Norwegian setting [2, 4, 10].

Change Management

The decision for change needs to be taken by the managers in response to patient safety and quality, and the leaders and policy makers at all levels need to be committed to the conducting of the process of change. Changing what is perceived to be a routine practice among health care workers may be challenging. Experienced health care workers feel secure in performing healthcare managements they are used to, and new protocols of care may face resistance [11]. Change management can be described under the following components:

Defining the Need for Change

The need for change in health care may originate from new research results, new methods or medication coming available, or from observed difference in complication rate between organizations or countries [12]. When a notable difference in quality of care between comparable organisations is identified, the organisation (maternity unit) should define a need for change in their current practice. Large differences in OASIS rates between countries and maternity units have been described

[6, 13–16], and these differences can be used to drive the need for change in maternity units with the highest OASIS rates [17].

Motivation and Resistance

Information relating to the need for change should be provided comprehensively to the clinicians (doctors and midwives) with a focus on the impact of the change on improving patient care and safety. Presenting a clear objective for the proposed change will motivate health care providers to accept the proposed change. Results from their own organisation should be presented in comparison to organisations with the best results (e.g. lowest OASIS rate). Clinicians' involvement is important to increase motivation, and getting key players and opinion leaders especially involved will increase the motivation of others. Practising clinicians should feel ownership for the planned change [12]. Resistance for change is common and should not be ignored. Listen to the arguments from those who disagree, arrange discussion groups for all employees, let everyone feel that they are heard. Common arguments against the change consist of genuine worries about the women's right to choose birth position and increasing use of episiotomy. Responses to these concerns should include evidence-based assurance that manually supporting the perineum does not need to increase the use of episiotomy. The woman can choose any birthing position she wants such as lateral, all fours, half-sitting, and in all these positions the midwife can reach the perineum with her hands. Indeed, when women are made aware of the importance of some birthing positions in reducing perineal trauma, they are willing to choose these positions during the last few minutes of birth.

Planning the Project

Identifying enthusiastic members of staff to drive a project where common practice is to be changed increases the possibility of success [12]. It is important to make a clear and practical plan with a specific time frame outlining when the project starts and ends, and ensure that staff are informed and fully aware of it. Choosing the responsible project leaders from amongst the enthusiastic clinicians and acquiring appropriate resources are essential to ensure the project has optimal managerial and financial infrastructures. To reflect the multidisciplinary nature of Maternity services, it is imperative to be inclusive of the entire maternity staff and to choose "experts" or "champions" among doctors and midwives, who are trained to perform the 'new' technique (MPP in this case). In our experience, an experienced independent trainer ensured that the MPP method was correctly learned and that it can be implemented in normal practice. Experience from the Norwegian projects reveal that three to four supervised deliveries are needed to for an experienced clinician to learn this method of MPP properly.

Implementing New Practice

Creating a practical plan to have everything in place when the project starts is important. When an experienced clinician trains "champions" to a high standard, they are then able to cascade this training to the rest of the staff. We propose that training should start with simulators. Training on birthing simulators can be performed in groups in defined timeslots, or continuously on the labour ward. Record names of all participants and keep this record visible, to show the progress of education among the staff. Training on simulators is needed to learn the method before entering the delivery room. Hands-on bedside guidance during delivery should also include the entire multidisciplinary team.

Evaluating Results

It is essential to set the baseline against which the impact of the improvement project will be measured. In this example, OASIS rate from the 1 to 2 years before the project started can be used as the baseline. When evaluating results during the ongoing project, one should avoid too short periods of assessment. For example, 1 month is probably too short a time period for evaluation (depending on the total number of deliveries), 3 months is a more adequate time period in most maternity units. Due to the fact that OASIS is a relatively rare event, large variation from month to month is fairly common.

Change That Does Not Work Out

Sometimes the results achieved as different from the expected ones. In this situation it is essential to undertake a thorough evaluation of the project to identify if there were any problems or mistakes. Is everyone trained? Has the education and training been appropriate? Is the method really used after training by auditing practice and OASIS case review? Continue with discussions and try to find out any residual barriers to implementation e.g. if using the method is difficult or if there is still resistance among the staff.

Maintaining Changed Clinical Practice

Throughout the project, new members of staff need to be trained to sustain the same level of improvement. Risk of regression amongst staff who have undergone the initial wave of training is not uncommon. Hence, continuous evaluation and refresher sessions of the training intervention are useful. Indeed, it may take years for the newly introduced clinical practice to become fully embedded routine practice. Therefore it is possible that the outcome of interest may continue to improve over a long time period even after completion of the quality improvement project.

References

1. Selecting Indicators for Patient Safety at the Health Systems Level in OECD Countries. 2004. http://www.oecd.org/dataoecd. p. 31–2.
2. Laine K, Pirhonen T, Rolland R, Pirhonen J. Decreasing the incidence of anal sphincter tears during delivery. Obstet Gynecol. 2008;111(5):1053–7.
3. Hals E, Øian P, Pirhonen T, Gissler M, Hjelle S, Nilsen EB, et al. A multicenter interventional program to reduce the incidence of anal sphincter tears. Obstet Gynecol. 2010 Oct;116(4): 901–8.
4. Laine K, Skjeldestad FE, Sandvik L, Staff AC. Incidence of obstetric anal sphincter injuries after training to protect the perineum: cohort study. BMJ Open. 2012;2:5. 10.1136/bmjopen-2012-001649. Print 2012.
5. Stedenfeldt M, Oian P, Gissler M, Blix E, Pirhonen J. Risk factors for obstetric anal sphincter injury after a successful multicentre interventional programme. BJOG. 2014;121(1):83–91.
6. Laine K, Rotvold W, Staff AC. Are obstetric anal sphincter ruptures preventable?- Large and consistent rupture rate variations between the Nordic countries and between delivery units in Norway. Acta Obstet Gynecol Scand. 2012;92(1):94–100.
7. Medisinsk fødselsregister M. The medical birth registry, Norwegian Institute of Public Health. n.d. Available at: www.mfr.no.
8. Leenskjold S, Hoj L, Pirhonen J. Manual protection of the perineum reduces the risk of obstetric anal sphincter ruptures. Dan Med J. 2015;62(5):A5075.
9. Basu M, Smith D, Edwards R, STOMP Project Team. Can the incidence of obstetric anal sphincter injury be reduced? The STOMP experience. Eur J Obstet Gynecol Reprod Biol. 2016;202:55–9.
10. Hals E, Øian P, Pirhonen T, Gissler M, Hjelle S, Nilsen EB, et al. A multicenter interventional program to reduce the incidence of anal sphincter tears. Obstet Gynecol. 2010;116(4):901–8.
11. Pirhonen T, Gissler M, Hartgill T, Pirhonen J. Experiences of expert midwives in a training program aimed at decreasing perineal tears. Int J Nurs MIdwifery. 2011;3(6):70–5.
12. Hewitt-Taylor J. Understanding & managing change in healthcare. A step-by-step guide. 1st ed. Palgrave Macmillan: Hampshier; 2013.
13. Pirhonen JP, Grenman SE, Haadem K, Gudmundsson S, Lindqvist P, Siihola S, et al. Frequency of anal sphincter rupture at delivery in Sweden and Finland – result of difference in manual help to the baby's head. Acta Obstet Gynecol Scand. 1998;77(10):974–7.
14. Räisänen S, Vehviläinen-Julkunen K, Gissler M, Heinonen S. High episiotomy rate protects from obstetric anal sphincter ruptures: a birth register-study on delivery intervention policies in Finland. Scand J Public Health. 2011;39(5):457–63.
15. Räisänen S, Vehviläinen-Julkunen K, Gissler M, Heinonen S. Up to seven-fold inter-hospital differences in obstetric anal sphincter injury rates – a birth register-based study in Finland. BMC Res Notes. 2010;3(1):345.
16. Gurol-Urganci I, Cromwell DA, Edozien LC, Mahmood TA, Adams EJ, Richmond DH, et al. Third- and fourth-degree perineal tears among primiparous women in England between 2000 and 2012: time trends and risk factors. BJOG. 2013;120(12):1516–25.
17. Bulchandani S, Watts E, Sucharitha A, Yates D, Ismail KM. Manual perineal support at the time of childbirth: a systematic review and meta-analysis. BJOG. 2015;122(9):1157–65.

Index

K.M.K. Ismail (ed.), *Perineal Trauma at Childbirth*,
DOI 10.1007/978-3-319-14860-1

MIX
Papier aus verantwortungsvollen Quellen
Paper from responsible sources
FSC® C105338

If you have any concerns about our products,
you can contact us on
ProductSafety@springernature.com

In case Publisher is established outside the EU,
the EU authorized representative is:
Springer Nature Customer Service Center GmbH
Europaplatz 3, 69115 Heidelberg, Germany

Printed by Libri Plureos GmbH
in Hamburg, Germany